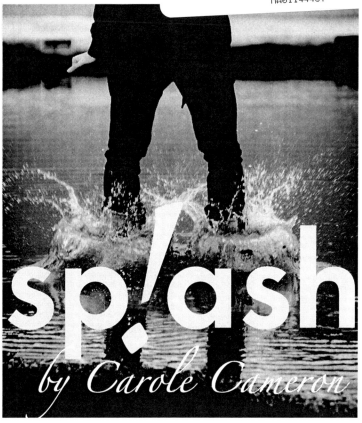

splash

by Carole Cameron

An introvert's guide
to being seen, heard
and remembered

Published by:

Career/LifeSkills Resources Inc
Concord, ON L4K 2M2
www.clsr.ca

Jacket Design By:

Capstone Communications Group
www.capstonecomm.com

Library and Archives Canada Cataloguing in Publication

Cameron, Carole, 1959-
    Splash : an introvert's guide to being seen, heard and remembered / Carole Cameron.

Includes bibliographical references.
ISBN 978-1-894422-50-5

    1. Self-actualization (Psychology). 2. Introversion. I. Title. II. Title: Splash.

BF637.S4C345 2009   158.1   C2009-904823-X

Table of Contents

Acknowledgements

Many thanks to all of those who offered me support, encouragement, insights, truths, connections, editing, coaching and humour.

Special thanks to Scott Campbell, Pamela Fennell, Paul Huschilt, Connie Maier, and Susanne Wussow.

Extra special thanks to all the generous introverts who supported my research through surveys, focus groups, interviews, and workshops. Your candid, personal, painful, joyful and thoroughly thoughtful stories and responses are a pleasure and privilege to share.

For James, thanks in so many ways for being exactly who you are.

Forward

I remember vividly my first meeting with Carole Cameron almost a decade ago. We met for coffee to discuss ideas about how she might grow her new business as a management development specialist. Carole's professional presence, enthusiasm, insightful questions and light-hearted demeanor combined to create quite a splash in my mind. I sensed immediately that this introvert and I would be good friends from that day forward.
This book is born out of lived experience. Whether in her previous work life as an HR professional and training manager for Nestle, in her current role as an entrepreneur running a very successful training business, or in her personal life with her many friends, Carole has demonstrated the effectiveness of the principles she describes in these pages. Carole consistently gets seen, heard and remembered.

My own experience as a trainer and coach has underscored the importance of the strategies and tactics she describes. Like Carole, I use personality type as a tool in many of my workshops to help people maximize the benefits of individual differences and minimize the frustration and misunderstandings they can create.

One of the frequent comments I hear from the introverts in my groups is that "It's an extravert's world." In many ways, they are right. Business tends to value and reward many behaviors which often come more naturally to the extravert. Rapidly responding in brainstorming sessions, schmoozing at networking events, speaking up frequently in meetings to promote one's ideas, and being "the life of the party" are just a few of the behaviours that come readily to most extraverts *and which get rewarded at work!*

Introverts often feel frustrated in group settings. Their potential contributions are frequently talked over by their louder extraverted colleagues. I have witnessed numerous times when an Introvert has said something two or three times during a discussion and then an extravert makes the very same suggestion in a much louder voice and everyone says, "What a great idea." All too often an introvert's insightful idea is ignored or even resented because it emerges through reflection well after the meeting is over and a decision has already been made (usually by an extravert who wants to move things along as quickly as possible). To then come back to the team and say, "I know we talked about this last time and decided to do such and such, but I have been thinking about it and I think instead we should…" is likely to be met with groans, grunts, and grimaces.

In the workshops where I teach the difference between introversion and extroversion, one of the activities I frequently include is to have the two groups separate and then answer a series of questions. One of those questions is, "What do you dislike about the opposite preference?" In separate groups, introverts discuss what they dislike about extraverts, while extraverts detail what they dislike about introverts. It is fascinating to watch the energy that exists in both groups as they hash out their dislikes of the other. Clearly, the extraversion-introversion polarity causes frustrations for all.

The groups then share their answers with each other. The typical list of what extraverts dislike about introverts includes:

- They are too quiet.
- They withhold important information.

- They take too long to give you the information.
- You have to pull things out of them.
- They are too serious.
- They seem distant and aloof.
- You can never tell what they're thinking.
- They come up with their ideas after we've already made a decision.

It's never easy to hear such criticisms, and I do my best to help mitigate the sting of such candid replies (don't forget the introverts have a chance to get even when it's their turn!), but it is important for each side of the dichotomy to see how their preference is perceived and experienced by the other. You may well think that these perceptions are unfair and that extraverts clearly don't understand introverts. And you would be correct.

But, like it or not, this is how introverts are commonly perceived.

So, what's an introvert to do?

You have two choices.

One is to commiserate with your fellow introverts and continue to feel frustrated.
The other is to act in ways that will ensure that you get noticed, heard and remembered.
The book you hold in your hands will give you an abundance of practical ideas that you can act on today to make sure that happens.

It is a great pleasure to introduce a book that I have watched grow from an idea in Carole's mind to its full expression in these pages. Read it, digest it, and practice it. You will soon find yourself making more of a splash than you ever could have imagined.

Scott Campbell, President & CEO
Personalities At Work

Section One:
Getting Your Feet Wet

Introduction

Making a splash doesn't necessarily require throwing a big rock.

Summertime for a city dwelling kid like me consisted of three glorious weeks of camping, travel and outdoorsy fun with my family, and then sweating it out for the rest of the time in the city. The neighbourhood kids spent the majority of summer hours at community pool, of course. I'll always remember the sights, sounds and smells of that pool. Invariably, every so often one loud and show-offy kid would venture to the high diving board, stand fearlessly at the very end, and look down to the crowds below, shouting "Hey, look at me!" Then he'd take a flying leap off the board, arms wrapped around knees, and land his "cannonball" with an enormous smack and a virtual tidal wave soaking the onlookers. Then he'd emerge with a huge smile, and repeat the performance. Kind of entertaining for a while, but it did get tiresome, and eventually the audience petered out.

One glorious, sweltering August afternoon, I caught a glimpse of a girl about my age (around 11 or so I guess) on her own at the other side of the pool, diving off the low board over and over again. She was perfecting her dive, a swan dive, my girlfriend now also watching, told me. The dive looked simple, effortless, graceful, and somehow perfect, although I knew nothing about competitive diving. As polished and perfect as her diving was, she certainly didn't draw a crowd. A few minutes later, she slipped out of the pool, towelled off, walked out the gate, hopped on her bike and rode away. I found out later that the girl was a competitive diver, and had won many medals in her age group.

Most kids at the pool, if asked later by their parents over the dinner table about their day, would remember the kid doing the cannonballs. Not many would have even noticed, much less remembered, the talented and graceful swan-diver at the other end of the pool.

Being Seen, Heard and Remembered

I am I said… to no one there…

One of the phrases I hear often from introverts which describes a huge frustration in their life experience is the feeling of being "invisible". Quite often the introvert has the right answer, or the perfect solution, or a great idea, but getting it out there for others to see is another story.

The thing I find most charming and endearing about introverts is that they don't "give it all away" at once. Getting to know an introvert is like peeling back the layers of an onion, or like digging for hidden treasure. The more you peel, the more you dig, the more you discover; and the more wonderful they can become.

Sometimes however, this does not work in the introvert's favour. As an introvert myself, I know that sometimes others in this extravert-dominant world just don't have the time or the inclination to dig or peel.

In the workplace, on the social scene, and in relationships, our success can rely on our ability to make an impression - a favourable impression. I call this being *seen, heard, and remembered.* We need to do the best job we can of making our "best stuff" visible so that we don't have to count on others to do some serious digging or to give us the benefit of the doubt. Why? Because let's face it, that won't always happen! And we can end up missing out on an experience, an opportunity, recognition, or a relationship by keeping our best stuff hidden.

The following exploration and strategies are drawn from the many experiences, stories and successes shared with me by the wonderful real-life introverts in my life and my workshops. There are some small and not-so-small things we can do to enhance our engagement with the world, to make an impact, to ensure we are noticed, to make a splash without hoisting a huge bolder over our head and heaving it into the pond. Remember the finesse involved in skipping stones? More like that.

What's So Different About *Splash*?

There is an endless array of books, CDs and workshops on the subjects of networking, image-making, and communication at our disposal. Many of them are very helpful. Subject matter experts in this field tend to be extraverts, and, not surprisingly, their content tends to suit those who share that orientation.

There is also a significant amount of material out there on the subjects of introversion, assertiveness, shyness etc. Some of you reading this book may have also covered some of this material. You have probably read about the inner workings of the brain and how mental processing is different for extraverts and introverts. You may have studied the phenomenological, empirical, and Jungian approaches to the experience of introversion, and their integration. You likely have taken the MBTI® Instrument, and/or some of the many other useful inventories to give you insights into the inner workings of your psyche and your personality. Most books out there on the subject of introversion offer a quickie assessment tool to help you determine whether you're an "innie" or an "outie".

Splash is different. In a number of ways:

It's written by an introvert (that's me) with input from other introverts (thank you) for introverts (that's you).

I assume you're pretty darn sure you're an introvert. We will take an individual focus: guide you through purposeful reflection on what you really want your life experience to be like, and what gets in the way, and offer practical tools and strategies that have worked well for other real-life introverts. It's about forming new habits that will help you create the life experiences that you want while remaining true to your authentic self.

Splash is not a "survival guide". Who wants to merely survive?! It's about taking control of your life, and making choices of behaviour that work for you and get you more of what you want. It's not about coddling yourself or buying into your own excuses. (Sorry!)

We'll look at 5 practical strategies and, within them, numerous techniques to help you be seen, heard, and remembered by the rest of the world. Specifically, we'll look at ways to:

1. Showcase your strengths,
2. Make memorable connections,
3. Create desirable first impressions,
4. Manage your energy, and
5. Make the big changes in your life.

A few years back, I read Jim Collins' book *Good to Great* because so many of my clients had been impressed with his message, and had started to transform their businesses by following the principles he uncovers. *Good to Great* is an awesome book. What I found particularly appealing was the fact that he and his research team didn't set out to prove a theory or create a new leadership or business model. They set out to discover what it was that made great companies (according to their specific definition) different from the rest. This made great sense to me, and added credibility to it all. So, I decided to adopt a similar approach to this project. *Splash* draws on the experiences, successes, and strategies of the introverts I've come in contact with in my business and my life. I gathered information and insights from hundreds of introverts (and a few errant extraverts) who were kind and interested enough to participate in my surveys and focus groups. What I'm sharing with you now is what they shared with me; about their "introverted experience" in the world, and the tools and strategies they've employed in order to enhance their careers, their relationships, and their life experience.

In short, the intent is to include enough background and success stories to make this book useful for you, provide lots of opportunity for reflection, leave out the boring bits, and focus on strategies that will work for you.

Creating the Life Experience You Really Want

What is success? Climbing the corporate ladder, finding the perfect mate, building a lucrative business, making a difference in the world? I see these not as measures of success, but as good examples of the wonderful and tangible by-products we can end up with by creating the life experience we really want. *Splash* is about creating a more enjoyable, engaged and satisfying existence in the world. Deliberately. Purposefully. Intentionally. It's a lot like running, or biking, or whatever you might do to keep fit and active. I don't get up at 6:30 am four times a week and run 5K because I like it, nor because it comes naturally to me. I do it because it brings to my life things that I value; accomplishment (hey, 5K might not impress you, but it sure works for me!) fitness, energy, and spending time outdoors. It also enables me to eat the fabulous food I love and have a glass or two of wine every so often! I do it deliberately, purposefully, intentionally. Many of the strategies we'll suggest in this book will not come naturally to you either. But let's face it, none us were born being able to ride a bike, make a soufflé, or speak Japanese either; these are things we learn.

I believe that when we are in a situation with which we are not completely satisfied, we have three choices:

1. grin and bear it,
2. improve it, or
3. change it completely.

Splash strategies fall into the second two options. These are about taking control, being in charge of your life, and getting what you really want.

Why I Felt Compelled to Jump In

I feel like I'm swimming upstream

There are a few compelling reasons that *Splash* came about: One was the understanding and freedom that came to me with the discovery of Carl Jung's "energy-based" definition of introversion, as I studied for my qualification to use the Myers-Briggs Type Indicator® (MBTI®), and Personality Dimensions®. My gosh, you mean it's NORMAL for about 33% of the population to focus their energy and attention inward rather than outward?? That "eureka" moment provided me the explanation for all those times I had felt like I was born on the wrong planet, and that everyone but me was engaged in a fascinating conversation.

As a kid and a teen I often felt like I didn't quite fit in. *Maybe* it was because my MBTI® type preferences are for INTJ (shared with only 3% of the rest of the planet, and most of them men). *Maybe* it was because until grade 11 I was about 6 inches taller than everyone else. *Maybe* it was because my mother wouldn't let me have Go-Go boots. I was never too sure…

I was thrilled to learn that there was actually an *explanation* for much of my awkward life experience, and that there were many others in the world who shared the very same experiences. My life didn't get any easier, but I had a certain level of understanding and acceptance. My life did get easier when I decided to take action to create my experience in life more like the way I wanted it to be.

The second reason I developed *Splash* is because I was fortunate enough to work for a number of years within a corporate culture that was fuelled by the belief that everyone has the potential to do great things. A positive, affirming, challenging environment driven by a talented, insightful, strengthening leader. I learned about personal accountability. That means no excuses! Instead of whining, complaining and blaming, our culture was rather to channel energy towards purposeful, positive action. (You may catch a ripple of this theme as we swim along together.) I learned first hand that you can change your life by changing what you believe. I learned that you can form new habits by raising your awareness of your behaviour, and making a deliberate choice to do things a different way.

Thirdly, *Splash* was born out of the frustration I experienced whenever I wanted to share my new-found understanding into introversion and others would say "What? You're not an introvert!" This response was likely based on the fact that I have what you might consider an extraverted profession, and that I am friendly and upbeat in my work and in my life. What people saw in my work was an energetic presentation, or lively workshop. What they didn't see was how long I prepared, how much I stressed over it, how much time I took to deliberately get psyched up for the performance. I repeatedly got annoyed and then got tired of trying to explain, prove and defend my introversion. So instead of simply continuing to be ticked off, I decided to put the energy to good use and design a program for others like me: **Introverts who are committed to getting what they want out of life, and stop missing out!**

Thus was born the *Splash* concept of becoming more fully engaged in the world and in our lives by finding ways to be *seen, heard and remembered*. As you share the *Splash* experience, you will:

- Review the misconceptions and refreshing realities about introverts and introversion;
- Consider what you'd like to be, do and have in your life;

- Reflect on and identify the behaviours, habits and excuses that get in your own way
- Explore the four varieties of introverts and their common experiences, challenges and success strategies;
- Learn five practical strategies for "making a Splash" to help you showcase your strengths, make connections, create desirable first impressions, manage your energy and make the big changes in your life; and
- Develop specific action plans to apply each strategy in ways that will work best for you.

Would the Extraverts Please Leave the Pool

I can't think if you're not listening

This book is not for extraverts. Its purpose is not to help extraverts understand introverts better (like *that's* going to happen!); Many of the things we cover, ideas we discuss, and exercises we do in our workshops would have the extraverts rolling in the aisles laughing at us. It's because they don't get it. Introversion is so outside of their own life experience we can't really expect them to do much more than understand the introvert experience on an intellectual level. Many of the skills we will work on developing, and habits we will start forming are things that tend to come quite naturally to the extravert. They don't really get that these behaviours sometimes require uncomfortable effort for us, or that we must actually do them quite deliberately. I expect that it all might sound quite ridiculous to them!

When the *Splash* concept was in its infancy and I began to enthusiastically tell my family, friends and colleagues about my fabulous idea to create a program on the topic of introversion and how to help introverts enhance their experience in the world, the introverts' eyes lit up! They expressed keen interest, they wanted to know more. The extraverts? I got rather puzzled looks from most, that kind of tilted head thing that dogs do, and not a whole lot of their natural enthusiasm. I began to confirm that my suspicions were correct, and that *Splash* could be a very unique and useful undertaking for a niche group.

In a nutshell, this book is not for extraverts because:

- they already have most of the books written with them in mind anyway,
- they may read something about extraverts that they don't want to hear, and
- they'd probably just laugh anyway.

Others Who Might Want to Consider Leaving the Pool

It's not for the feint of heart, but it just may be great for you.

The **Splash** experience just may not be for you if you are negative, needy, co-dependent, resigned to failure, flakey, the king or queen of excuses, closed minded, not willing to get a little uncomfortable, fatalistic, or if you think Dr. Phil and Judge Judy are just big meanies.

It's kind of "boot camp for introverts", and it could be for you if you are eager and ready to do the work to create a life that is more the way you'd like it to be!

About Introversion

"Others don't seem to understand it's a state of being, not a state of doing."
Ruby Childs

Misconceptions and Misunderstandings; Belly Flops and Getting Sand Kicked in Your Face

In my workshops, these are some of the most common responses I hear from introverts about how they believe they are perceived. See if some of these sound familiar to you:

quiet	shy	private
aloof	snobbish	reserved
lacking confidence	dislike people	loners
can't interact	like boring things	low self-esteem
no sense of humour	disdainful	lacking ideas
unsociable	party-poopers	dull
guarded	withholding	timid
withdrawn	arrogant	non-team players

We know that these labels aren't exactly accurate, and we also know that introverts can be dreadfully misjudged and under-estimated.

Kathie, an introvert, holds a senior position in marketing with a large multi-national company. She has created a very successful career, however not without discomfort. She also possesses a lovely wry sense of humour. Kathie writes: "I think there are very negative perceptions about introverts – that they are complete loners who can't interact with people – and are potentially not very likable. Also that they can't be leaders, can't be funny, aren't warm, and that they don't belong in marketing."

How Do Others See Me?

"There is no reality, only perception." Dr. Phil McGraw

Jot down a few thoughts on how you believe you are sometimes misread, misinterpreted or misunderstood. Be specific. Which people do you believe perceive you this way? In which circumstances does this happen?

i am sometimes perceived as:	By whom?	Under what circumstances?

The Extraverts Get a Word In (What a Surprise)

Perhaps even more interesting and relevant is that the descriptors that the introverts offer up are actually very similar to the (negative) responses we hear from extraverts about how they perceive introverts. **NOTE**: Extraverts do also report positive perceptions of introverts, more on that good news later.

Here's an important revelation I got from an extravert's point of view: While working on this book, I came up with what I thought was a very clever (although unflattering) remark about extraverts: "Extraverts don't actually expect us to hold up our end of the conversation, they just don't want to get bored in-between their own stories." I ran this nasty extravert-bashing comment by my extraverted friend Scott for his input. His response was "We do expect you to hold up your end of the conversation. When you don't, we interpret it as boredom, apathy, indifference, or lack of intelligence about the topic". Whoops! Good information to have.

So Why Is It Important To Know How We Are Perceived?

Why can't you just love me the way I am?

As introverts we are often misread by others. So, what's the big deal? Why should we go out of our way to do something about it? These misinterpretations only become important if they get in the way. In the way of what? Of reaching the personal and professional successes we dream of, and the experiences, opportunities, recognition or relationships that we want! We may have missed out on some of these things because we haven't gone out of our way to learn new habits and skills that will facilitate us in being who we want, doing what we want, and having what we want.

In the early days of my corporate career, as I moved up in the Training and Development world, I began to get feedback indicating that others thought I tended to "tune out" in meetings. I would sometimes appear to be deep in thought, making no connections with those around me. Of course, what I was doing was generating ideas, and mulling them over in my head so they'd sound at least half-cooked when I spoke them aloud. Meanwhile, the extraverts were busy thinking out loud, appearing to be full to the brim with ingenious solutions and ideas. I realized that if I was to be perceived as a competent, enthusiastic, valuable player on this team, that I need to play a little differently. So I, painfully at first, began to practice the fine art of thinking out loud, and as time went on, it became more and more comfortable. The result? All of a sudden I was "creative and brilliant" in my colleagues' and boss' eyes. Worth the effort? Definitely!

Acknowledging that we need to do something differently, or learn new skills or strengthen certain abilities with practice is not an admission of failure. Learning new habits and skills will simply get us more of the wins that we want.

What I really don't want is to give all the power of how I am perceived over to anyone else! I want to be the one more in charge of what others see and believe of me.

The Confidence/Self-Esteem Thing

"Extroverts appear to be confident, just as introverts appear to be good listeners."
Carole Cameron

This is perhaps the most limiting misconception about introverts and introversion. Introversion is not really about confidence, but it can sure look like it. In reality, there are certainly many confident introverts in the world, just as there are many insecure extraverts.

Extraverting tends to look like confidence. Bold, loud, and sure. What does "confident introversion" look like? A confident introvert is completely comfortable with speaking less and listening more, with not blurting out ideas as they come to mind, with thinking a little longer on a point. They have no compelling need to show the world all the great stuff they've got in there. Well, that's just dandy from a healthy ego point of view, but what does that look like to the rest of the world? In this predominantly extraverted world, this behaviour does not really come across as confidence. Yes, you are confident, and acting authentically, but it doesn't get you very far towards being *seen, heard or remembered*! Or towards getting the things that you say you want in your life.

Let's face it, in the real world, perception is reality. In Section Two, strategies 1 – Wear the Suit that Shows Your Best Stuff and 3 – Do Your Best Drive First, focus on deliberately creating a more outward demonstration of our inner confidence, and making sure no one misses seeing our best stuff.

It is also important to note that introverts do not hold the exclusive rights to being misinterpreted, misunderstood or misread. Extraverts can be misinterpreted as poor listeners, self-centred, egotistical or bossy. (But somehow they don't seem to fret about it too much…)

It's All About Energy

I'm not anti-social, I'm just selective with my energy.

For those of you well-informed, card-carrying introverts, you know one fundamental, indisputable, basic truth: IT'S ABOUT ENERGY. Simply put, the source of an introvert's energy is internal, and they tend to focus their energy inwardly as well. An extravert is just the opposite. They draw energy from outside themselves, and focus it there too.

The terms introversion and extroversion were introduced by Carl Jung. In his 1921 book, *Psychological Types* he elaborately outlined the concepts. (If you can last until page 285 that is; only then does he get to the really exciting 'type' stuff.)

When left to their natural devices, introverts:

- are more reflective than expressive
- are more likely to respond than to initiate
- tend to think first, and talk second
- tend to talk less and listen more

For most introverts, we have a finite well of energy. Sometimes it drains rather suddenly, and when its dry, the party's over. Time to cut the conversation short and leave the yackety crowd behind. Almost like an energy switch.

I have owned my own management and training consulting firm for over 8 years. Before that, I worked for 15 years in the corporate arena in Human Resources, and Training and Development. Lots and lots of time spent in front of people, in meetings and in the classroom, being witty, engaging and energetic. It's all very doable, it's just pretty darn tiring for an introvert. I want and need to seriously "recharge" after a day of highly energized interaction. My extraverted colleagues tell me that they are <u>energized</u> by classroom time! Wouldn't that be nice!

Terry, a facilitator and pastor shared his experience with me: "I noticed that it took me a lot more time to get emotionally ready to facilitate or preach than other colleagues. I thought I was in the wrong career since it was so much more work! Once I realized that introverts just naturally need more time to re-energize after an extraverted activity, I realized I was not a "loser", I just need to plan more gearing up time and down/solo time."

Depending on whose statistics you choose to believe, the extraversion / introversion split in North America is around 70% / 30%. Here's another take on the same statistic that I rather like, sited by education experts Jill D. Burruss and Lisa Kaenzig: "Introverts are a minority in the regular population but a majority in the gifted population."

Also important to note is that introversion is not the same as shyness. Introverts choose solitary over social activities by preference, whereas shy people avoid social encounters out of fear. And, as counter-intuitive as it may seem, there are shy extraverts!

"I don't want to belong to any club that will accept people like me as a member."
Groucho Marx

One more distinctive quality of this book is that there is no set of qualifying questions to help you determine if you are an introvert or not. I sincerely doubt that an extrovert would pick up this book in the first place. But just for fun, check out the Splash test...

The *Splash* Test

Ok, so we know that you know that you're a true blue, bona fide, genuine, card-carrying introvert. You know this because more than a few of the following statements describe your life experience to a tee:

- You can hardly wait for the party to be over so you can go home.
- While away on business, you would rather have your own hotel room, instead of bunking with a chatty colleague even though it doubles your cost.
- You would rather drive the 500 km alone to an out of town wedding instead of sharing a ride with "strangers".
- You use email and put off making a phone call until you absolutely have to.
- You are convinced that you've "already had this conversation" but you haven't.
- Your best arguments, rebuttals and comebacks come to you half an hour after you need them.
- You don't see why solitary confinement is a punishment.
- At a corporate event where you know few people, you are in agony, and it takes all your strength not to flee.
- You've used your children as an escape strategy (I'd better get going now, James needs to get to hockey practice/finish a project/eat dinner...).
- After an extroverted activity out of town, you want to go to your room and order room service, while the rest of the gang wants to go out dancing.
- You feel more connected without a cell phone.
- You don't get how two extraverted people can think they're having a conversation, it looks to you like a series of interruptions.
- Before making an important phone call you make notes and rehearse what you're going to say.
- You turn down the enthusiastic offers of a new acquaintance to hang out because you already have four perfectly good friends, and you really don't need any more.
- Your idea of a great vacation is a week by yourself with a stack of books.
- You believe that networking is way over-rated.
- At the movie theatre, your extraverted friends refer to the person sitting by themselves as that "poor lonely soul" and you're thinking they have the best seat in the house.

- At a conference, you present brilliantly in front of 1200 people but leave the room a few minutes into the social hour.
- As a kid your mother kept telling you to "go out and play with the kids on the street" when you were quite happy in your room with your Barbies or trucks.
- You broke up with your girlfriend or boyfriend using a post-it note.
- You think people with 297 friends on Facebook are superficial.
- You're not sure what they mean by "an awkward silence".

Refreshing Realities

"Introverts are taking over the world...quietly."   Paul Huschilt, Humourist

Alright. So we know what it is, and we know that's what we are. And here's the good news about introversion:

Refreshing Reality 1 - There are many happy, well-adjusted, satisfied and successful introverts in the world!

Famous people:

My all-time favourite musician is Carly Simon, whose song writing, recording and performing career spans 4 decades. Carly's "stage fright" is well known. She has given us countless memorable songs that have touched our lives.

Johnny Carson (OK, now I'm really dating myself), the warm, well loved and funny host of "the Tonight Show" for 30 years.

Barack Obama, at the time of publishing the newly elected President of the United States brought calm, hope, and decisive action to a nation in need. Suddenly being smart, classy, and quietly thoughtful became trendy.

Actors: Meryl Streep, Clint Eastwood, Glenn Close, Kevin Kline, Diane Keaton, Anthony Hopkins, Tom Hanks, Laura Linney, Johnny Depp. Need I say more?

How about the elegant Jacqueline Kennedy Onassis, the outrageously humourous Mark Twain, the charismatic Pierre Elliott Trudeau? Or the brilliantly logical Mr. Spock, the child prodigy pianist Schroeder, the handsome "Professor" on Gilligan's Island, the gentle philosopher/theologian Linus van Pelt with his endearing blue security blanket.

OK, on we go before we get really silly.

Not-so-famous people:

We all know very dynamic and successful introverted colleagues in many walks of life, including in those we tend to think of as "extraverted" professions. Some of my talented introverted colleagues include:

Craig in real estate sales and management; Susan in sales, marketing and training; Scott a mountain climber, university professor, public speaker and experiential trainer; Catherine who runs a successful marketing and web-design company.

Who do you know? Think of the fabulous introverts you admire, who are happy, successful, and seem to have figured it out.

_____

_____

_____

Could you have a conversation with some or all of them to learn their success strategies?

Refreshing Reality 2 - Sometimes assumptions about introverts work in our favour!

"Let a fool hold his tongue and he will pass for a sage." Pubilius Syrus

Here are some of the good news stories that introverts have told us:

> "It creates the impression that I'm a "deep thinker", a stable presence, and a credible resource."

> "In business, introverts do not seem to have the need to seek approval from others. Super extraverted behaviour can give the appearance of insecurity and unprofessionalism."

> "I have many more repeat clients than one-offs. This is a good thing from a business perspective. It's because my clients trust me, and I've taken the time to establish a one-on-one relationship with them."

And from the extraverts:

> "Introverts don't seem to embarrass themselves like we do."

"Introverts are fabulous listeners."

"Introverts are better "readers" of people, they take the time to observe and think."

"On our team, it's the introverts who provide the focus and bring us back on track."

"Our boss is an introvert. He provides a very calming effect on our hectic, stressful department."

"Introverts have thought things through by the time they share an idea. By then it's a pretty good one. We listen to them seriously."

"Our best customer service reps are introverts. They take the time to actually listen to the customer's needs. This is what customers want, not to be entertained."

Refreshing Reality 3 - Introverts, like fine wine, get better with age.

We are only young once, after that we need some other excuse.

As we move on through our lives, learn new skills, widen our scope of experience, and see and do more things, we are better able to put life's events into perspective. We become more comfortable in our own skin. We get to be seen as wise, losing many of our inhibitions and fears. We gain courage based on our successes. Extraverts become more reflective, while introverts become more comfortable expressing who they really are and what they really feel.

Refreshing Reality 4 - We truly like extraverts, we just don't necessarily want to BE one.

I'm OK, you're OK - in small doses.

Introverts don't want to become extraverted just as vegetarians don't want to learn to eat meat. They really and truly don't want to be the kid doing the cannonball thing. We want to be winning the swan dive competition, but darn it, no one's paying attention. Everybody just happens to be down at the end of the pool watching the cannonball kid.

"I love extraverts, many of my friends are extraverted. They're more fun! But I don't want to hang out with them all the time."

"I would like to be able to turn on the extraversion when necessary, but I wouldn't want to have to stay like that all the time."

Most introverts tell us that even if given a magic wand, they wouldn't use their wish to become an extravert. Mainly, they enjoy their life experience, *but do not enjoy what they feel they are missing out on.*

There's no denying that we would enjoy having some of the things that we perceive extraverts to have:

- Conversing with ease
- Always having something to say "on the spot"
- Being the initiator
- Establishing relationships with ease
- Being known by others
- Being remembered by others
- Add your own here: _____

Why do they call them extraverts… do they have something extra?

Carl Jung's original theory suggested that we are all born with a natural home-base location somewhere along the extraversion/introversion continuum. He suggested that we could enjoy the best life experience if we develop the ability to slide up and down the continuum with ease as required. I think this is the ideal skill to work on developing. It's not about becoming an extravert. It's about sliding along the scale at the right moment to the place that gets us where we want to go. That's making a splash!

About You

"He who looks outside dreams, he who looks inside awakens." Chinese Proverb

Before we launch into the strategies that will help you be *seen, heard and remembered*, it's time to focus on you. Who are you? Who aren't you? What do you really want to be, do or have in your life? And what *specifically* gets in your way? Once you've had a chance to answer these questions, you can review the strategies in the next section with more focus.

About Being Authentic

Being me, only better.

Sometimes what gets in the way of doing something differently is the thought that changing how we do things will compromise our authenticity. Authenticity does not mean that we can't or shouldn't adapt to the needs and demands of a particular situation. It means accepting who we really are without rigidity. Flexibility in the moment is not phoniness, it's being skilful. One of the things that separates humans from the rest of the animal kingdom is that we have much more choice over our actions rather than simply responding to our instincts. Adapting to the moment is a way to honour who we are as human beings.

In her work on psychological type and temperament Dr. Linda Berens describes the nature of our temperament as dynamic, not static; influencing, not limiting. Dr. Berens describes our personality with a model of "3 selves"; the Core Self, the Contextual Self, and the Developed Self. She contends that we come into the world with a predisposition: our Core Self. We are free to behave in situations in a variety of ways. This is our Contextual Self. Our temperament pattern will influence which skills we are drawn to develop and which ones we develop more easily. These become our talents. We can, and do develop skills to deal with the many situations that life brings us. Over time, these skills become prized assets of our Developed Self.

I want to become more comfortable being uncomfortable

The more we repeat behaviours that are Contextual, the more comfortable and skilled we become. They then become part of our Developed self and take far less energy and conscious attention. While these behaviours will never energize us the way that acting out of our Core self will, they are extremely useful and far less taxing when they are highly developed.

Notice the part about the **energy**? Thought so. Anyway, all that to say, 'Please don't play the "authentic" card on yourself and sabotage what you originally set out to do by opening this book!'

What Colour is Your Bathing Suit?

Or, introverts come in 4 delicious varieties.

Although we introverts share many qualities, preferences, tendencies and misgivings, there is no denying that each of us is a unique individual. Much of the work that I do in my business makes use of psychological type and temperament. You may be familiar with these models of personality. You may have used the tools or inventories that help us determine where we fit into the models; the MBTI®, which distinguishes between 16 separate 'Personality Types', or True Colors®, and Personality Dimensions®, which identify 4 'temperaments'. (This is by no means an exhaustive list.)

We're going to use the temperament model to dig a little deeper into the different kinds of introverts that are swimming along with us.

So, briefly, what is temperament?

Stephen Montgomery puts it cleverly in his book People Patterns: A Modern Guide to the Four Temperaments. "Temperament is an inherent personal style, a predisposition that forms the basis of all our natural inclinations; what we think and feel, what we want and need, what we say and do. In other words, temperament is the inborn, ingrained, factory-installed, God-given, hard-wired base of our personality," he writes. Temperament is born of the many forefathers of personality and personality type, including Carl Jung, Isabel Briggs Myers and Katharine Cook Briggs, and David Keirsey. Actually, the idea that human beings come in four basic models has been around for a very long time; we see "quadrant" theories in the works of Plato, Aristotle, and Hippocrates.

Personality Dimensions® is one of the most widely used tools in this area, which to provides an easily understood methodology for building self-awareness, self-esteem and effective communication strategies. The names we'll use for the four temperaments are from Personality Dimensions: "Resourceful Orange," "Organized Gold," "Authentic Blue" and "Inquiring Green". It's important to note that both introverts and extraverts come in the same four varieties. So we also share many behavioural similarities with those extraverts who share our temperament colour!

The following summaries come from many existing written sources, and, most valuably, from the real-life introverts who participated in our workshops, interviews and surveys.

The *Resourceful Orange* Introvert

These folks are most at home in the concrete world; with things that can be seen, touched and used. They have keen senses, love working with their hands, are born for action, and for making free, spontaneous manoeuvres that get quick, effective results. They have a natural talent for the arts, they typically are painters, musicians, actors, athletes, politicians, salespeople, and may be attracted to "action" type careers such as firefighters, racing car drivers, and pilots.

Core Psychological Needs: Freedom to act on the needs of the moment, the ability to make an impact now

Talents: Seeing and seizing an opportunity, adapting to the circumstances, troubleshooting, pragmatic problem solving, managing a crisis, creating options

Stressors: Constraint, boredom, no opportunity to make an impact

When I'm out of energy: Can display a "don't mess with me" attitude

As an introvert I sometimes feel like I'm missing out on: Opportunities to do things or have fun.

The *Inquiring Green* Introvert

This gang gives much importance to intellect and proficiency. They thirst for knowledge, and seek to know the foundations and principles behind why things are as they are and how things work. They don't generally care about being politically correct, efficiency is more important. They have a burning desire to achieve their goals. They work tirelessly, and pride themselves on the ingenuity they bring to their work. They are the engineers, the professors, the scientists, and the systems people.

Core Psychological Needs: Knowledge and competence, mastery and self-control

Talents: Strategy, systematizing, inventing, envisioning multiple possibilities, using words precisely, classifying, abstract thought, long-term thinking

Stressors: Powerlessness, incompetence, redundancy, lack of knowledge

When I'm out of energy: May become intolerant and impatient. "I'm surrounded by idiots"

As an introvert I sometimes feel like I'm missing out on: Being seen as knowledgeable or competent

The Authentic Blue Introvert

These individuals are passionate about personal growth, and nurturing harmonious relationships. They believe that life is full of unknown possibilities and untapped potentials. Highly ethical in their actions, they hold themselves to a strict standard of personal integrity. They are the very soul of kindness. Particularly in the closest relationships, they are filled with love; and they cherish warm intimate friendships. They gravitate to jobs as counsellors, teachers, ministers and advocates.

Core Psychological Needs: Meaning and significance, unique identity and purpose

Talents: Diplomacy, empathy, seeing and developing potential in others, imagining better futures, seeing ethical issues, advocating for causes or others

Stressors: Insincerity, betrayal, lack of integrity

When I'm out of energy: Can become down, less optimistic and idealistic, can appear "plastic", e.g. like faking concern for others

As an introvert I sometimes feel like I'm missing out on: Quality of relationships

The Organized Gold Introvert

These are sensible, down-to-earth people who are the backbone of institutions and the true stabilizers of society. They believe in following the rules and cooperating with authorities. They believe that in the long run loyalty, discipline and teamwork get the job done right. They are careful about schedules, cautious about change, and take pride in being trustworthy, hardworking and reliable. You'll find them in nursing, teaching, accounting, management, administration and police work.

Core Psychological Needs: Responsibility, duty, sense of belonging

Talents: Logistics, supervising and monitoring, measuring, providing for others' needs, warning of danger, developing policy and procedures, maintaining and passing on traditions

Stressors: Abandonment, lack of discipline, insubordination, irresponsibility

When I'm out of energy: May withdraw from responsibility, complain, sigh

As an introvert I sometimes feel like I'm missing out on: being appreciated and acknowledged for all that I do

So What Colour is Your Bathing Suit?

Read over the descriptions for each "colour". Tick off the items that seem to describe you.

Which colour is most like you? _____

Second most like you? _____

Least like you? _____

Knowing your temperament pattern can go a long way to understanding yourself and others better, and in our case, can help you choose the best strategies which will work most effectively for you on your journey to making a splash in your own life. The differences in the four temperaments also can explain why not all of the strategies and tools we'll introduce in Section 2 will be equally appealing to you.

What You'd Really Like to Be Do or Have

Down to the short strokes

In these two sections we're going to take a good honest look at the things that are really working well in your life, and the things that you'd like to add, change, improve or just darn well get rid of. You will set some specific goals that you want to achieve. We'll also look at some of the things that you are doing, saying and thinking which could be getting in your own way. This will provide more clarity, focus and context for reviewing the strategies in Part Two and for selecting the ones which will work best for you.

As you work through the following exercise, think specifically about the aspects within each category which you believe are affected, influenced or limited by your preference for introversion. (Rather than another factor which might be unrelated, or outside your control.)

Carve out a chunk of time where you can focus on this reflection without interruption. Find a comfortable place. Some people do their best reflection in a comfy chair, some at their desk, some lying down. You may want to start by making notes, you may want to start just by closing your eyes and tuning in to each category.

Take plenty of time. I suggest focusing in on one life area completely, thoroughly, thoughtfully before moving on to the next. Don't feel like you have to do it all at once. You may even want to run your reflections by a trusted friend. This may help you to be more precise in your responses. Ask them not to comment or advise you, but rather to ask some probing questions for clarity and specificity.

Don't limit yourself to what you believe is reasonable or realistic. We'll get to that later. Think about what would you change, add, improve or eliminate.

Jump in. See you on the other side!

Reflection Exercise:

How's it Going? What's Working, What's Not?

What would I change, add, improve or eliminate?…

	Just super-duper, thanks very much!	Something different that would be nice	Something different that would be FABULOUS
Lovelife/Romance/ Marriage/Sexlife			
Parenting			
Career			
Social			
Spiritual			
Health and Wellness			

Envisioning the Other Shore; Setting *Splash* Objectives

Aim at nothing and you'll hit it every time

The time has come to narrow things down and get focussed. It's not wise, as well as it's next to impossible, to work on everything all at once! (On the other hand, there is no doubt that once you begin to form new habits and behaviours, new things will begin to happen in all areas of your life.)

Review the reflection exercise you've just completed. If you could pick just 3 things that you want to be significantly different in your life, what are they? Be as specific as possible. For example, rather than saying "I want to get noticed at work", say "I want my ideas to be acknowledged and praised by Chris Roberts". Rather than "I want to improve my business", say "I want to increase my client base by 25% this year". Rather than "I want to improve my relationship with my partner", try "I want to show my partner how much I care for her in ways that are meaningful to her".

You get the idea.

My Top Three *Splash* Objectives:

1. _____
   _____

2. _____
   _____

3. _____
   _____

Be sure to keep these top of mind as we head through the strategies in Section Two.

Just one more thing to do before we dive right in. In the name of thoroughness, we'll do a bit of a reality check. Just one more look in the mirror, I promise, then you can step out of the change-room and start swimming.

Am I Getting in My Own Way?

"The first principle is that you must not fool yourself – and you are the easiest person to fool." Richard Feynman

You may feel you were born swimming upstream just by virtue of being born an introvert. You may think that you have to work harder than others to get what you want out of life. You also may be getting in your own way. You may be doing, saying or thinking things that just do not help you get where you really want to go. In **Splash** terms, we call these *cement shoes*. *Cement shoes* are things we say and do and think that get in our way, weigh us down and can even pull us right under.

Cement Shoes

"Nobody can make you feel inferior without your consent." Eleanor Roosevelt

Cement shoes is a term we've come to know from gangster movies and TV shows like The Sopranos. You know, the mobster "takes care of" the aggravating fellow by having him stand in a box of wet cement until it dries, and then tosses him in the river. The weight keeps him under, and he ends up "sleeping with the fishes".

I use the term to mean the things that weigh us down, pull us under, keep us from getting or being what we want, but the difference is that it isn't usually a mobster that puts them on us. We do it to ourselves, whether we are aware of it or not.

For example, I know that most of my extraverted clients prefer the telephone over email. I know that the phone is the best way to reach them or to get a response from them. Yet, more often than not, I find myself defaulting to email, because it's more comfortable for *me*. The result? I get to stay comfortable, but I miss building the client relationship in the most effective way, which is critical for the growth and sustainability of my business. And, in many cases I have not used my time effectively.

Have you ever been lucky enough to end up the same room as a person that would be a truly advantageous contact for your work or life in some way, but you held back on initiating a conversation? The result? A missed opportunity.

You know what I'm talking about. Let's take a look ....

1. Things I Know That I Do or Say Which Get in My Own Way

_____

_____

_____

_____

_____

How this limits me in getting what I say I really want:

_____

_____

_____

_____

_____

2. Our *cement shoes* are sometimes things that we are not even aware of! Sometimes our behaviour, or choice of words or body language is sending a message that we do not intend to be sending. (Remember all those misconceptions?)

Sometimes *cement shoes* are more about how we make others feel when they're around us. Here's what some extraverted folks have noted about introverts:

> "I feel like I have the whole weight of the conversation on my shoulders."
> "He speaks so slowly, and with so many pauses, it makes me fidgety!"
> "I would like to get more of an immediate reaction or feedback."
> "Something about her body language makes me think that she's dying to get away from me."

It certainly can be the case (for introverts and extroverts alike) that we are sending messages that we do not intend.

Feedback is a very powerful thing. In my Presentation Skills workshops we include an option to video tape each speaker. For those of you who've had the opportunity to see yourself making a presentation on camera, you know what a valuable (and sometimes humbling) experience it is. It's an amazing opportunity to see yourself doing things and sounding in ways that you might never have imagined! I remember my first go at it. I imagine I'd see a smiling, light-hearted confident me on the silver screen. No such luck. The woman I saw was super serious and seriously slouching! All that to say, feedback is a good thing.

Comfort Zone Warning!

This next exercise may not be the most feel-good assignment that you've ever done, but the feedback will be extraordinarily valuable if you choose to give it a go. This exercise is going to take more leg-work than the last. And courage. Your assignment is to get feedback. Feedback about yourself. Your mission is to discover some of the things that you do or say *which you are not yet aware of* that could be getting in your way.

Hmmm, Who Should I Ask? What Should I Ask Them?

Ask people you trust will give you an honest response. Ask people you trust period. Try to get feedback from an assortment of people in your life; colleagues, friends, family, those who've known you a long time, and a shorter time. Don't ask people who you suspect have just been itching to tell you what's wrong with you and what you should be doing about it. (You know who I mean...)

Come from a position of personal and professional growth, rather than from the position of lack or unfulfillment. Start off by positioning it something like this:

> "I'm currently working on...
>
>> a. achieving a certain goal
>> b. getting a new job
>> c. taking on a new responsibility
>> d. insert your own

...and I would like to polish my image in order to ensure my success. I'm trying to get really clear on how I come across to other people. So I'd like to ask you a few questions, and would appreciate your most candid and honest responses."

Then get into the nitty gritty. Here are some example questions you could use:

- "Where I'm going, I need to come across as very approachable. How would you rate me as far as being approachable? Why?" Ask for specifics.
- "I have had feedback that I don't look too comfortable in a (certain type of) situation. Would you agree? What makes you say that?"
- "There are certain things that I've already identified to buff up, like smiling more, and making more eye contact with clients. Is there anything else that you would suggest?"
- "What was your first impression of me? Why?"

You get the idea. So hitch up your suit, put on your nose plugs and go for it! You can record the summary of your findings here:

Things I Didn't Know That I Do or Say Which Get in My Own Way

_____

_____

_____

_____

_____

How this limits me in getting what I say I really want:

_____

_____

_____

_____

_____

3. And finally, sometimes the *cement shoes* we craft for ourselves are on the inside. Things that we tell ourselves, or false beliefs. (These could also be from an external source and we've internalized it.) I have heard this voice referred to as our inner critic, the demon inside, the gerbil on the wheel, the little voice inside your head, etc. You know what I mean. And if you are thinking "Nah, I don't have a voice inside my head", well, *that's* the voice inside your head. Self-talk is very powerful, so we need to be very tuned into what we are saying to ourselves, and very deliberate about what we choose to say!

This inner voice can keep us stuck where we are, and worse. The good news is that on the flip side, this voice can help us dramatically change our life experience, if we get it to switch over to be a cheerleader for our team
Some of the less than helpful messages we send ourselves could be:

> "I'd never be able to do that!"
> "I'm not funny enough to pull that off"
> "That's just not my style"
> "I never can remember people's names"
> "I never can think of anything to say"
> "If I do a really good job I will get recognized eventually"
> "These extraverts are such jerks"

OK, one more time, let's take a look. This time, on the inside…

Things I Tell Myself That Get in My Own Way

_____

_____

_____

_____

_____

How this limits me in getting what I say I really want:

_____

_____

_____

_____

_____

Hopefully, you are now equipped with insights, and focussed on the *Splash* goals you have set for yourself.

Let's jump in!

Section Two: Making a Splash! Strategies and Applications

The Game Plan for Making a Splash

Time to drop your towel and get in the water!

So you've now had a few good opportunities to reflect on who you are, where you are, and what you'd *really* like to be, do, or have in your life. Great work! It's time to start taking action.

We're going to look at *Splash* strategies within five different areas:

1. Showcasing your strengths.
2. Making memorable connections.
3. Creating desired first impressions.
4. Managing your energy.
5. Making the BIG changes in your life.

Note that not all strategies and tools will suit you or your specific objectives in making a splash, but don't let yourself use this as an excuse for not trying something that just might bring you success if you give it a fair shot.

Many of the strategies we'll discuss are what you might call simple. (More choice words might be used by our extraverted friends for sure!). As you'll see, simple is probably an accurate descriptor in many cases. BUT! Who said that simple = easy? For example, changing a light bulb is simple, but it's not easy when it's 20 feet up in the air. Smiling and making eye contact is simple, but it's not easy when you are totally drained of energy. Introducing yourself to a stranger is simple, but it's certainly not easy when you feel invisible.

Two things to remember as we swim through this portion of the book, where you will commit to trying new things that will make your life more the way you want it:

1. **It's not supposed to be easy.**

2. **It gets easier.**

If it were easy, everybody would do it.

A good friend and colleague of mine also owns and runs a successful business, and we often commiserate about the joys and rewards of working in this way. We also share our stories about the challenges, frustrations, the time and dedication required. He likes to say: "well, if it were easy, everybody would be doing it!" A good reminder that it does take hard work and commitment to get great results in our lives and our work. It's not supposed to be easy!

It gets easier.

With the acquisition of any new skill or talent, one classic learning model tells us that we progress through four stages of competence:

- Unconscious Incompetence (we don't even know yet that we can't do it)
- Conscious Incompetence (we are aware that we don't do it very well)
- Conscious Competence (we see that we are good at it, but it takes a lot of concentration)
- Unconscious Competence. (doing it well has become second nature)

Of course the desired state is unconscious competence, where we have truly developed a new skill, created a new habit of behaviour which becomes now just part of how we do things.

We may not always evolve all the way to this ideal. At the very least, as we practice, engage new strategies deliberately, and develop new behaviours and habits, we will expend less energy and experience less and less grief, terror and anxiety than we did for starters.

Let me give you an example:

My personal trainer, Pat, is a very competent, intelligent, caring, introverted woman. She tells about her transition from a traditional career in banking into one that truly engaged her and allowed her to meet her core need to help others reach their full potential. "Being "trained" to become a personal trainer was wonderful" she says. "I love to learn, and the whole field of health and wellness totally matches my values. I learned about anatomy, biomechanics, muscle structure and function, and behaviour modification techniques. I passed exams with flying colours. But when the time came to actually work one-on-one with clients, I was terrified! I knew exactly what to do, but felt so uncomfortable at first, and I experienced huge anxiety before meeting with each one. I was able in most cases, to "psych myself up" and appear to be positive, energetic, directive and supportive, but it was totally exhausting! I completely loved my new career, but I lost a lot of sleep in those early days! As time went on, the more I worked to develop my skills, my "act" as a confident, competent trainer was no longer an act. Pat had reached unconscious competence through lots and lots of practice and successful experiences.

I felt much the same when embarking on the *Splash* project. I was compelled to make the book, the workshop and the coaching happen, but I still felt terrified of some of the "extraverted" activities which are necessary to make such a project successful and far-reaching. Think book tours, radio and tv interviews, yikes!

Author Susan Jeffers coined the fabulous phrase "feel the fear and do it anyway".

We may not ever get to a place of complete comfort, but with continued practice and increasing competence, we can lessen the anxiety we experience around any particular activity or behaviour, and we can expend less energy doing it and stressing about it.

Start by causing a ripple, then move towards making a splash*!*

Within each section you'll have opportunities to examine ways to put a number of strategies into practice in your world. We'll do this on two levels; the first to allow you to check it out, in smaller, safer ways, and the second to really forge new habits that will get you where you want to go.

Application Level One: "Testing the Waters"
Think of these as things which you can do in smaller chunks, not too risky, a chance to pretend, practice, see what happens and how it feels.

Application Level Two: "Diving Right In"
These are the things that are more challenging for you, more risky; maybe doing Level One things when you really don't feel like it, or when you're out of gas, things that really require you to "get psyched up" for them, and happily recover from afterwards.

Everybody ready? Take a deep breath, here we go.

Splash Strategy 1 - Wear the Suit That Shows Your Best Stuff

Toot your own horn (more like a whistle, not an air horn!)

We all can think back through our lives and remember some of our favourite clothes. Maybe a comfy pair of jeans, maybe a favourite t-shirt. Sometimes we wore things until they were threadbare because we got feedback like "wow, that blue shirt really looks great on you", "that sweater shows off your green eyes", or "you look like a million bucks in that outfit". This strategy is about doing just that – uncovering a bit, and showing the world our best stuff – on purpose!

My partner Doug is a larger-than-life extravert. He's overflowing with positive energy, ideas, stories, solutions, questions, information, opinions. When he walks into a room, he fills it. There's never any trouble seeing, hearing, or remembering him! He's my hero and my inspiration. I often feel like we possess many of the same great characteristics; positive energy, great ideas, inspired thought, problem solving ability, insight…. but _mine_ tend to be on the inside. Right where the world can't see them.

Frederica Balzano's book _Why Should Extroverts Make All the Money_ is a very useful guide to job search and networking. In it she states "I have found that many introverts are so confident that someone is going to recognize their greatness that they don't even try to increase their exposure". (So much for lack of confidence!) Well folks, that's just not the way it really works, is it? Unless we get really lucky. Personally, I'm not prepared to leave it up to someone else to notice me. So I coach introverts to get more comfortable with "tooting their own horn", or at least making it easier for others to see their strengths and talents.

There is a lot of good material out there about "personal branding". Much of this is written by extraverts, for extraverts. Lots of bold statements and loud rah! rah! rah! We'll take a similar approach, but one that I believe is more palatable for introverts.

Showing Your Best Stuff

What this means is

1. identifying what your strengths, talents, abilities and gifts are,
2. clarifying just how you want the world to experience and remember you, and
3. committing to trying some strategies which can move you in the direction of your choice.

Once Again, It is About Remaining Authentic…

Some things just don't fit. I can cram my size 10 feet into a size 8.5 shoe, but it sure doesn't feel very good. Nor is it good for the health of my feet! I once tried to cram my INTJ independent, introverted, unconventional self into a "Leaside Soccer Mom" costume, but that didn't fit either. Years ago, I read John Gray's *Men are From Mars, Women are From Venus.* Although I know that this book helped a great number of people, (it does fit about 75% of the population), I found it stereotypical, and ill-fitting for me. Why? I didn't fit the target audience. I was a "thinking" woman with a "feeling" male partner, so I just took the male/female advice, reversed it, and used the bits that seemed helpful and useful. What's the moral of the story? If it doesn't fit, don't buy it, or don't buy into it. Take the bits that *do* fit, (or could fit with a little effort) and make them work for you.

Showing your best stuff is about doing the most with what you've got. You may remember having your "colours done"; this process identified which colours to wear in order to bring out the best in your skin tone and hair colour. There is also a science with respect to body shapes; this is about dressing in ways that make the most of your assets and minimize your not so great body parts. These are both about the importance of being aware, educated and deliberate!

A **Splash** survey participant, William, shared with us: "I'm 6'2", 275 lbs, with a voice that is deep, warm and weathered. I'm a retired naval officer with a commanding presence – nobody ever fails to notice, or remember me." Now that's showing your best stuff!

The following exercises and reflections will help you identify the great stuff you have to show the rest of the world, and to narrow down the things that will make you most memorable to others. It will involve reflection and also getting input from others. Hint: This is not the day to be humble!

EXERCISE #1

What is My Best Stuff?

Southern belle Scarlett O'Hara was known for her seventeen-inch waist. We remember Princess Diana's shy smile and her passionate support of numerous social causes. Jackie Kennedy is the picture of elegance, cultivation, intelligence and innate sense of style. Albert Einstein's theory of relativity and unique hair stylings make him memorable. What is memorable, special, or striking about you?

Physical Appearance: What is distinctive about your appearance? (Think: very tall, very short, red hair, flair for fashion, gap in your front teeth, very fit, great calves, naturally wavy hair, big bright eyes, sexy voice…)	
Knowledge and Expertise: What do you know better than most? (Think: areas where you are a subject matter expert, specialized technical knowledge, speak 5 languages, know how mechanical things work, movie trivia buff…)	
Talents and Abilities: What can you do better than most? (Think: innate ability to read a situation, run marathons, photographic memory, can fix machinery and cars in a flash, musically talented, put people instantly at ease…)	
What do others tell you they like or appreciate about you?	
What do you love? What brings out your passion, and sparks your energy?	
What do you want to be remembered for? How would you like others to describe you? What do you want others to know and remember the most about you?	

Well done. Now look it over again. Be sure you haven't sort-changed yourself, and that you have asked at least 6 other people for input, preferably from the different parts of your life.

What is My BEST Best Stuff?

Now we make a short list. Of the fabulous stuff you identified about yourself above, which are the best of the best? Select either none, one or two from each category.

Physical appearance	
Knowledge and expertise	
Talents and abilities	
What do others like or appreciate about you?	
What you love and get passionate about?	
What do you really want to be known and remembered for?	

EXERCISE #3

How Do I Showcase My Best Stuff?

Now we get to work! Be creative and courageous here. This is the part where we figure out how to make your best stuff seen, heard, and remembered by the rest of the world!

Let's start at the beginning with your physical appearance. Write down the memorable characteristics you identified above, and then let's think about splashing them up. Remember, Level One application strategies are not too risky, give you a chance to pretend, practice, see how it feels and what happens. Level Two application strategies are more challenging, maybe more risky, uncomfortable or tiring.

My Best Stuff: **Physical Appearance**	*Splash* Application Level One: Testing the Waters	*Splash* Application Level Two: Diving Right In
Example: Beautiful smile	• Make a deliberate point of smiling more. • Look people in the eye and even without saying anything, smile at them. • Create secret reminders to myself to remember to smile.	• Smile at people even when I'm tired and grouchy.

My Best Stuff: **Knowledge and Expertise**	*Splash* Application Level One: Testing the Waters	*Splash* Application Level Two: Diving Right In
Example: Advanced knowledge in the use of MS Office applications	• Make presentations using spectacular and impactful visuals. • Provide data in reports using advanced macros.	• Volunteer to run a seminar for folks at work who would most benefit from this knowledge.

My Best Stuff: **Talents and Abilities**	*Splash* Application Level One: Testing the Waters	*Splash* Application Level Two: Diving Right In
Example: Run marathons	• Mention to others that you are getting up very early these days because you are in training. • Tell others that you are competing this weekend • Post the picture of you crossing the finish line at your desk.	• Use running/training analogies in your work presentations. • If it's a fund-raiser, ask 10 different people than usual for sponsorship • Hang a medal at your desk.

My Best Stuff: **What Others Like of Appreciate about Me**	*Splash* Application Level One: Testing the Waters	*Splash* Application Level Two: Diving Right In
Example: I help others focus in on the real issue at hand.	• Rather than just stating what is obvious to you, showcase your insight with a preface like "The issue clearly is a complex one. What we want to get at today is x and the real concern to overcome is y. Let's focus on that."	• Do Level One when I am really not in the mood, or when I'm completely out of steam, tired of the extraverts' babbling. • Toot your own horn a bit by saying "you know, I've been told that the greatest value I bring to meetings like this is helping the group focus in on the real issue at hand. So that's what I'd like to do now..."

My Best Stuff: **What You Love and Get Passionate About**	*Splash* Application Level One: Testing the Waters	*Splash* Application Level Two: Diving Right In
Example: Fine Wine	• Mention the wine-tasting class you are teaching. • Use wine-making metaphors in your work presentations (as people know more about you, they'll ask you questions, giving you an opportunity to painlessly show your passion and knowledge on the topic). • Organize a road trip to a winery. Invite colleagues and/or clients. Talk knowledgeably and ask smart questions at the wine tasting bar.	• Invite your workmates, or some folks at the club, or people you'd like to get to know to come to a fun wine-tasting event at your home. Get a friend who's brilliant with food to take care of that end so you can focus. • Write a simple book like "Wine 101", or "Fine Wines for Under $15". Talk about it as you write it, and as it comes out.

My Best Stuff: **What Do You Really What to be Known and Remembered For?**	*Splash* Application Level One: Testing the Waters	*Splash* Application Level Two: Diving Right In
Example: My writing abilities and clever sense of humour	• Submit articles to the company newsletter	• Submit articles to association newsletters, and trade journals, and send the link to colleagues who would share an interest in the topic. • Say yes when they ask you to speak to their group.

Now *that* was a lot of work! And, a lot of things to try to do all at once! So let's get focussed. Go back to page 24 and review your 3 top *Splash* objectives. Then review the ideas you came up with in this section, Show Your Best Stuff, and select 2-3 actions that will best help you achieve your *Splash* goals, and that you can commit to start doing right now. Be as specific as possible; when, where, and with whom.

My Best Stuff:	How I'm Going to Showcase It:

Carole-Anne talks about showing some of her best stuff: "I am very articulate and that is a quality that is noteworthy. I work at developing that, and like to find opportunities to express myself. I enjoy making an impression with the clothing that I choose to wear as well. I tend to be iconoclastic and I share my views when I have the opportunity. I have developed a good sense of humour. I value being unique, non-conventional and a bit eccentric. People remember me for it."

Splash Strategy 2 - Swim to the Other Side of the Pool

"I am a part of all that I have met." Alfred Lord Tennyson

When it comes to making connections with others, we know that introverts are more naturally inclined to respond rather than to initiate contact. Introverts are much more likely to answer a question when asked, than to ask it. We also know that the opposite is true for extraverts!

The reality is that you can't expect others to see, hear or remember you if they don't know you, or know you're there! What many of our workshop participants tell us is that without being willing or comfortable to initiate connections with others, they know that they miss out on many enjoyable relationships, exchanges and experiences with others.

A few years ago I was on a business trip to Chicago. I arrived well on time at the airport, and sat on my own, reading, as we waited to board. We all boarded on time, and again, once in my seat, I pulled out my book and began to read, thus successfully avoiding having to make silly small talk with my neighbour. Well, as does happen, there was a delay in take-off. And then another. And then another. In the end, because of some kind of a maintenance issue, we were all asked to de-plane and wait in the terminal for another aircraft. So once again I chose a seat on my own, and continued reading. By this time I had been completely self-contained for about 5 hours. I must admit I was getting bored with my own company. I looked around, and saw a group of women sitting at a table having a few snacks together. So I summoned up my courage, walked over to the table, selected the most approachable looking one, and asked if I could join them. What followed was a lively conversation, a few glasses of wine, a new business association and a lasting friendship with a delightful woman, Catherine. A big lesson for me. There can be a huge payoff if you make a little effort.

So Strategy 2 focuses on making connections with others. On purpose.

Listed below are 9 strategies for making more and better connections with others. They won't all be appealing to you, and some will be more challenging than others. Review them, and as you do, start thinking about "Would I do this? Could I do this? Where, when and with whom would this work? Where, when and with whom am I willing to give it a try?"

Then we'll summarize and create your action plan at the end.

1. Provide a Reason for Others to Initiate Contact

This one comes from Helen, a very talented and creative marketing specialist. Here's an example: at a conference or professional event, you can be the one with the supplementary handout, or serving the wine, or working the registration table. This puts you in the more comfortable position of responding vs. initiating, and also gives you the opportunity to show how articulate and knowledgeable you are. And show off your great smile.

Another classic technique to provide a reason for others to initiate contact is to sport a "splasher". A splasher is anything you carry or wear that is unique or unusual. It could be a colourful handkerchief, a glitzy broach, an interesting addition to your name tag, a funky pair of shoes, a school ring (a Superbowl ring also works well if you have one.). It provides something for others to notice and to comment on if they want to make contact with you. Of course you will want to become a "splasher watcher" too, giving you a perfect opener if you decide to initiate contact. "Excuse me, I couldn't help noticing your lovely amethyst earrings. Is your birthday in February like mine?"

2. Use the Phone
Extraverts like it better, and will tend to check and respond to voice messages sooner than to the carefully crafted emails introverts prefer. This can be a challenging shift in behaviour, but well worth the effort. If you need to think first, clarify what you want to say, make a few notes, fine. That's what I do! Ruby shares that she has chosen to do this very intentionally at work. "I've made a new habit to not hide behind emails, but as much as possible, to pick up the phone instead, or even to go and speak with the person face to face."

3. Speed Up
Walk a little faster. Talk a little faster. And while you are at it, talk a little louder too! (Not all the time; try it in bursts, especially when someone's watching!) Act as if you are a high energy person. Walk briskly across the room, or across the street or up the stairs. Act as if you have somewhere important to go and you are looking forward to getting there.

Be prepared to hop about from topic to topic if you're conversing with an extravert. Be responsive, add short, enthusiastic comments like: "No kidding!" "Wow, I never thought about it that way!" "Why did you do that?" "Well isn't that interesting!" Speak loudly and clearly when you need to. And don't worry too much about interrupting an extravert, it's all part of the rhythm.

4. Have Your Answers Prepared
We are inevitably faced with the dreaded question "So what's new and exciting?" (Don't you hate it when all those interesting things you've done in the last month somehow just fly out of your head?) Put some thought into your response in advance. Do what extraverts do – embellish it! I so admire extraverts for having responses at the ready which sound so seamlessly unplanned. The key to getting the same spontaneous effect for introverts is to plan or even practice ahead of time. Here are some ideas:

<u>Splash up your hometown:</u>
At a business function or conference, you will invariably be asked where you are from. Have a few clever responses at the ready which will then give them something else to comment on. For example: "Well I'm originally from Atlanta, which you may have guessed from my accent, but now I live in the Big Apple" or "I'm from Brantford Ontario, the hometown of Wayne Gretzky". Or "I lived in big bad Toronto all my life, and I've recently moved to the country, which I am totally enjoying…"

<u>Splash up your job:</u>
Another question to anticipate both social and business contexts is "What do you do for a living?" Again, give your conversation partner something to work with by positioning what you do for a living in a unique way. For example; instead of saying "I'm a training consultant" (who knows what the heck that means anyway), I say "I teach management teams to get better results from their employees" If I'm feeling very brave, I might even add "One of the interesting assignments I'm on right now is with a client who manufactures kitty litter!" So instead of saying "I work in a clothing store", try "I help people select clothes that best suit their body type, and help them create the image they're going for."

So what is "new and exciting"?

Before a social event or business function, or a day at work, make a mental note of things that you'd like to bring up in response to that inevitable question. Ask yourself: what books/articles have you read? what movies/plays/seminars have you seen? did you get a new car/boat/home/pet/job/client recently? took or are planning a vacation? mastered your PVR? finally broke down and got a Blackberry? did something for the first time, (cooked a turkey) or learned something new (how to drive a standard transmission)?

5. Psych Yourself Up (Pre-Energizing!)

If it's stupid but it works, it isn't stupid.

One of my favourite clients, Carol, is a fun-loving, fast-paced extravert. I need to match her energy. When I'm preparing for a call to her, I get the key objective of my call very clear in my mind. I determine what my approach will be, and I come up with a punchy opening comment or question to start with. OK, here comes the goofy part. Then I energize myself by jumping up and down a few times, or making some noise like clapping my hands or a drum roll on my desk, and call her from a standing position. Try it sometime. I bet you will notice a difference.

As you head into a meeting, phone call, function, or party, tell yourself you're going to give it all the energy you've got for x minutes, and then leave. This way you can focus your energy wisely and also know that it won't have to last forever. You're in control!

6. Turn On Their Tap

Just get the extraverts started. Be friendly and approachable. Ask a couple of great open-ended questions about them. Any extravert worth his salt will run with it and talk and talk and talk! I love to tap into the extravert's wonderful energy this way. (The trick is to get energized, not exhausted!). Here are a few:

> "Did you catch the game last night?"
> "I've been admiring your purse/tie/watch/haircut, where did you get it?"
> "Do you think we'll all be swept away in this rain storm?"
> "I love this warm weather, it's such a welcome change from the snow in my hometown at this time of year"
> "What did you think of the keynote speaker?"
> "I enjoyed my salmon at dinner, what did you have?"
> "How do you spend your free time?"

Do what extraverts believe we are good at, listen! And occasionally make an encouraging comment. In some cases people will wind up thinking you're a fascinating person because in your presence they find themselves saying fascinating things! Now that's memorable!

Let's hear that again...

Here's a good trick to get others talking, (and it can also be used as a way to create a diversion so you can slip away). In a group of colleagues, in a lull in conversation, say "Mark, I bet everyone would love to hear what you just told me about... your latest success with... what you just discovered about... the time you... Just be sure that this allows your colleague to make a splash themselves (don't pick the time they got drunk and embarrassed themselves, fell off their bike, or bungled the account.)

7. Be Congruent and Look Approachable

Be very aware of what your body is "saying". Are your words and your body language in synch? Our body language can sometimes scream out messages we think nobody can hear. Sometimes, after a full day, you are feeling "I'm tired, please don't notice me or talk to me, I just don't have the energy to deal with you" and guess what, that's what your body language is saying too. Sure, sometimes it is just best to disappear. But if you wouldn't mind making a few friends or a new contact by investing a short period of time, then let your body language say so.

Looking approachable goes a long way towards initiating contact. Rather than standing by the door or sitting down when most are standing, move closer to where the action is. Create a reason to "travel'. The food table, the bar, a display on the other side of the room, and as you move through the crowd make lots of eye contact, and smile. Be aware of your body language; lots more about this in Strategy 3 about making first impressions.

One of the exercises I do in workshops helps participants practice this. (Oh yeah, this is one of the things we do which would have the extraverts doubled over with laughter.) To say "make lots of eye contact" is easy. To do it consistently and deliberately, for many introverts requires practice! So I have the group wander around in an open area of the classroom, and when they approach another, they are to simply make good eye contact, smile, and say a loud "Hello!" The homework assignment is to take a morning walk. As they greet others on the street, they are to smile, make eye contact and give up a big "Good Morning!". Practicing on strangers is great non-threatening fun!

Listen to your voice mail greeting. What does it say about you? Try splashing it up! Prepare something energetic and friendly. Write it down. Then before you record it, rehearse it out loud. (Yes, really) Stand up and say it clearly and a little louder than normal. Then record it. Listen to it again. What do you think? Get some feedback from others too. I get lots of unsolicited feedback on my greeting. "I love hearing your greeting, so upbeat and energized". All I did was do it on purpose. And yes, I wrote it down, rehearsed it, and recorded it standing up.

8. Act Like a Human Bean
When I was a kid, for a while I mistakenly thought that the phrase "human being" was actually "human bean". ("Hey Mom, the guy on the tv said that this is really important news for all human beans. What are they?")

What I'm getting at here is a couple of things. Being human, fallible, imperfect can be very endearing to others. Self-disclosure, sharing something about yourself opens up so many opportunities for others to know you better, (think memorable) and to chime in (think connection).

- Smile or laugh at a joke even if it's not the funniest, and what you really want to do is roll your eyes.
- If someone shares an embarrassing moment, be willing to admit you've done the same thing, and tell about it.
- Be responsive if someone jokes or teases you, even if you are almost at the point of bolting from the event.

Everything in context
I hope it goes unsaid that you will want to choose your moments to be endearingly imperfect! For example, admitting that you are a hopeless speller is not going to go over too well when you're chatting with your boss and her colleagues. You get the idea.

9. Offer to Help Someone

"We cannot hold a torch to light another's path without brightening our own."
Ben Sweetland

What a gracious and feel-good way to make a connection. It can be as simple as offering to open the door for a colleague whose hands are full, or offer some advice/counsel in your area of expertise to someone in your referral network. Kindness is memorable.

My Action Plan
Lots of ideas to consider. As you've read along, you've probably been thinking things like "Wow, great idea" and "How idiotic" and "I could do that one." So, let's sort it out. Review your thoughts and notes from the 9 techniques above. Write down what you feel might work for you, or that you'd be willing to give a go. Be very specific. What exactly would you be willing to do, and with whom, or in which situations. Don't worry about filling in every square. Just make a note of the best, most likely strategies for you.

"Swim to the Other Side" Making Connections	Yes, I could try this. With whom, in which situations?
1. Provide A Reason For Others To Initiate Contact	
2. Use The Phone	
3. Speed Up	
4. Have Your Answers Prepared	
5. Psych Yourself Up (Pre-energizing!)	
6. Turn on Their Tap	

7. **Be Congruent and Look Approachable**	
8. **Act Like a Human Bean**	
9. **Offer to Help Someone**	

Now let's focus. Make a shorter list of the items above. Which actions do you feel would make the biggest impact on you getting what you say you want?

Are they application Level One: "Testing the Waters" (things which you can do in smaller chunks, not too risky, a chance to pretend, practice, see how it feels and what happens)? Or are they more like Level Two: "Diving Right In" (things that will be more challenging for you, more risky; more tiring)? What makes them tougher? Summarize your plan below.

My Connections Strategies:

_____

_____

_____

_____

_____

Leona shared with me her wonderful **Splash** success story: "My first paying job was as a cashier at a pizza restaurant many years ago. I was very shy and introverted but I HAD to talk to people. To make things easier I started to look for the unusual. As people came up to the counter I would look for anything that would catch my eye so I could genuinely comment on it. I found that people appreciated that I noticed their beautiful scarf, or that they looked very happy and content after their meal or they had a beautiful brooch on or whatever. The other thing that helped me was to look at the colour of the person's eyes. This helped me get comfortable with eye contact! As I slowly gained confidence at work I then decided I would try to make everyone I came into contact with smile. These things felt very awkward at first and I have to confess that I felt very foolish at times! But so be it! I now have no trouble connecting with strangers."

Splash Strategy 3 - Do Your Best Dive First

"It is only shallow people who do not judge by appearances." Oscar Wilde

You are engaged to speak at an event sponsored by your professional association. You prepare well, and your impression is that your presentation was engaging, informative, and humourous, although it did run a little longer than planned. The feedback sheets indicate that the presentation was a little dull, too long, and the jokes weren't funny.

You are at your wife's Christmas party, attended by her work colleagues and their spouses. When you arrive, everyone seems to be engaged in lively conversation. You try your best to connect with a few people, but nothing takes off and more than a few of them excuse themselves from your company after a minute or so to "refresh their drink." You figure that all these people know each other well, and you are just a newcomer. You find out later that most of them had just met that night.

You are excited to be invited to make a proposal to a new client. You create a fabulous presentation and deliver it well. You believe that you were able to establish a good rapport with the client at the meeting. You are later informed that you didn't get the contract because the client did not feel a strong enough connection with you, in order to feel comfortable working with you and trusting of your work.

Do any of these scenarios sound familiar? Of course. Experiences like these occur all the time. Without knowing, you are leaving an impression with others that a) you are unaware of and/or b) you did not intend to.

Why are these impressions we make on others when we first meet them so important? Psychological research shows that people give credence to and remember initial information much more readily than later information. Although at first sight, people only see a tiny sampling of you, to them it represents 100% of what they know of you! Then they tend to try to fit whatever subsequent information that shows up into our first impression. First impressions are difficult to reverse or undo.

Think about others in your life, and when you first encountered them. What was your first impression of them? Has your first impression changed much? If not, perhaps you are a great judge of character, or perhaps you are just normal like the rest of us. We have a natural tendency to seek out or be more aware of information that is consistent with their first impression. Oh, it's good to be right!

Depending on which expert you ask, it takes only three to seven seconds to make a first impression. They say that just over 50% of that impression is based on your appearance, your body language, your facial expressions, your mannerisms, and how you are dressed. About 40% of a first impression is based on the sound of your voice and the quality of your speech, and a mere 5% is based on what you actually say. (Hmm, maybe not such bad news for we of few words!)

Halos and Horns/Angelfish and Devil Rays

Another thing that "human beans" do is make assumptions and generalizations about another based on positive or negative traits. For example, it's been shown that someone who appears positive and upbeat is also assumed to be successful, intelligent and likeable. This is called the "halo effect". On the flip side is the "horns effect". For example, someone who appears to have nothing to say can also be perceived as boring, aloof or not so bright.

So what does this mean for introverts with so much of our best stuff packed up on the inside? We've already talked about how easy it is for introverts to give the wrong impression. And if we look back at what so many of you have told us, it's usually because of our body language, and perceived approachability and interest.

We've talked about showing your best stuff in Strategy 1. Showing your best stuff is especially critical right up front, where those important first impressions are taking place. This is when we can do our most important work towards being seen, heard and remembered; for the moment, and for the times ahead.

A Peek in the Reflection Pool

Part 1
So how do others see you upon first impression? (when you're not completely invisible, that is) Do you know? Does it depend on your energy level that day? Jot down some descriptors of the first impression you think others get of you:

_____

_____

_____

Part 2
Find as many trusted colleagues, family and friends as you can and ask them what their first impressions of you were:

_____

_____

_____

Part 3

What is the first impression that you want to make on others?

_____

_____

_____

Part 4

What's working? Where are the gaps between the impression you'd like to make and the impression you're making? Why are there gaps (what do you think you are you doing or not doing)?

_____

_____

_____

Filling in the Gaps

Alright, your work is done for now. We'll spend the rest of this chapter looking at some strategies to move you ahead as far as making your desired first impression. Then we'll revisit your goals, and decide on which strategies you will try on for size.

The first strategy is by far the most important. Most important to making a memorable first impression, to showcasing your strengths, to making great connections, to dealing with obstacles and challenges that will come your way, and to creating the life experience that you want. What is it? I call it...

1. Your Take on the Lake

"A positive attitude converts a personality that is easy to ignore into one that isn't."
From Learning to Lead by Pat Hein and Elwood. N. Chapman

OK gang, time to take a little breather. Put your feet up, take a sip of wine. I'd like you to take a moment, and think about all the people in your life that you really like to spend time with. Those who enrich your life, make you laugh, make you think. It feels like home in their presence, it was always worth the time spent with them, you look forward to seeing them. Now think about the reasons you feel that way about them. I'd put money on the likelihood that you consider these people in your life to be "positive" people. Not the ones who bring you down and suck the energy out of you. You know who those ones are too.

What feels like about a million years ago I used to watch Richard Simmons on TV. He is an upbeat, energetic little fitness and wellness personality who was incredibly popular at the time. I even bought one of his VHS workout tapes to use at home. There's a line he used at the end of that video that has never left me. He said, among other profundities, "Surround yourself with positive people." I've never forgotten that sentiment. And as years went by, I realized that in order to surround myself with positive people, I had to be positive too, or else they weren't going to be too interested for too long.

Truly positive people just won't get sucked into other people's misery. They don't stick around for too long at a pity party. They don't participate in gossip, looking for fault in others, complaining, blaming others. They focus on what can be done rather than what can't. They focus on making things happen rather than moaning about what will never happen.

Once I figured this out, I began to make a conscious effort to "feed myself" with positive literature, books, tapes and activities. I call this "get your $#*! together" stuff. And I also began to spend less and less time with those people in my life who didn't rate well on the positivity/negativity scale.

An important element within the "get your $#*! together" stuff is often referred to as personal accountability. This is about being totally accountable for the things that come your way in life. Not that you *caused* them, necessarily, but to be responsible for dealing with them in a way that works out best. It's about being in control rather than being a victim. It's also being expectant that good things are coming your way. You can call this silly if you want but I always fully expect to find a good parking spot, or find a good deal at the book store, or find a kumquat at the grocery store. And it always happens. Well almost always. This is my simplified version of "The Secret".

Another reason I feel so strongly about this power of positive thinking stuff is because the alternative is so darn unappealing! Imagine walking around expecting bad things to happen. And then when they do, feeling powerless to do anything about it. As the old rhyme goes,

> *"Two men look out of prison bars*
> *One sees mud, the other sees stars."*

I cannot possibly write or talk about the power of a positive attitude without mentioning my mom. Catherine is unstoppable, unsinkable, she is deliberately and purposefully optimistic. At 81 she is more energetic, interesting and joyful than many young people I know. And I'm thankful that she has been such a great role model for me.

Before I have to re-name this book *The Power of Positive Thinking* (although I'm pretty sure someone already claimed that one) I'd better wrap up the rant, and just summarize by saying that if you really want a more joyous, engaged, positive life experience, your best bet is to truly put a positive spin on things, and surround yourself with people who do the same. Allow the law of attraction to kick in.

"My point... and I do have one." Ellen DeGeneres

Ah yes, we were talking about first impressions. What's the connection? If you truly embrace a positive attitude and deliberately let it show, it will shine through to others the moment they meet you. A genuine positive attitude is attractive, infectious and memorable.

If you'd like to do some deeper work in this area, there are many many wonderful resources out there. At the end of this book I've listed some of my favourite authors on the topic.

2. The Stories Your Body is Telling

Our body language, to a great degree, can tell others what we're thinking, feeling, if or if not to approach us, what we might be like, whether we're telling the truth or lying. Of course, this could be either accurate or inaccurate information! Not that that matters, because we know that perception is reality. I like to tell this story in workshops:

My son James played hockey at a competitive level for many years when he was younger. As a result, we spent lots and lots of time together in the car, driving to and from various arenas. One particular time, my hands were on the wheel but my mind was elsewhere, grinding through a challenging situation at work. James said to me "Mom, why are you angry?" Brought back from my fog, I said "Pardon?" He repeated "Why are you angry?" I said "I'm not angry, James". To which he replied "Well you should tell your face!" I was completely unaware of what my face was "doing", which had sent an incorrect message.

We talked a little earlier about temperament, and Personality Dimensions®. I am an Inquiring Green. I happen to have a natural inclination when I'm thinking, as do a few others who share my colour, to break eye contact, and look upward and to the right. (By the way, that's where all the answers to Trivial Pursuit questions are!) And if I'm speaking with a client, and thinking at the same time, I might speak not looking at them, but looking into that magical corner of the room. What is my body telling them? I have a googly eye? I'm talking to my imaginary friend? What would you think? Thank goodness a client-who-became-friend gave me the invaluable feedback that this is what I tend to do! Very good to know. It's like someone being kind enough to tell you that you have spinach in your teeth.

The point is that we need to be very very aware of what our faces, bodies, hands, and legs do naturally, and to temper those movements with ones that match our intended message. So much of any kind of personal development is about raising awareness in order to make more deliberate choices. And so is this. So as far as first impressions go, what do you want to choose to do deliberately with your body? Here are some suggestions. Check them out. As long as your own individual charm and style have a chance to shine through, you'll make a splash.

Smile More
This one is a magical charm. If you are a natural smiler, great! Notch it up even more. If you tend to have a less than happy look on your fact when you are in "neutral", become more purposefully aware of what your face is doing at any given time. Go out of your way to give a lovely natural smile to people when you're talking with them, when you pass them on the street, or in the hall, or in the gym. It could be a wide, toothy grin, or a charming upturn of the corners of your mouth. I dare you! You'll see what happens! Smiling gives others the impression that you are positive, approachable and interested.

Posture
I inherited the tall gene from my parents. As child, and particularly as a teenager, I was very aware that I was quite a bit taller than most others my age. I developed a slouch, and a weird kind of way of standing with my hip sticking out, I suppose to bring me more in line with others. Ok, with the boys. These were habits I needed to break, and I did, once I came to embrace and enjoy my height.

Great posture is a simple way to instantly look more confident, knowledgeable, and physically attractive. Keep your shoulders down and back. Practice standing up straight, head held high and walking briskly with purpose. Swing those arms, too. Poof! You're much more noticeable and memorable.

Take Up Space
As an introvert, you have probably at some time or another experienced the sense of feeling invisible. Susanne tells a terrific story about this. She was in a gift shop, waiting to pay for her purchases at the counter. The shopkeeper seemed not to notice her, and went along serving everyone else. Susanne shares, "I decided to make myself visible by 'inflating my physical presence'. I took a deep breath, straightened up, squared my shoulders, raised my chin and radiated my unhappiness with being ignored. It seems I somehow mystically materialized into the shop, and I got the service I was looking for!"

Taking up space means just that. Becoming "larger" in every sense of the word. This is a technique I coach on particularly for making presentations or speaking to a group. You can take up more space by moving around the room, using larger gestures, animating your facial expressions, speaking a little louder, and punctuating your speech with emphasis on certain words. An exercise we do in workshops emphasizes the point. Each participant is given a short phrase to deliver. For example "The team's performance this quarter has far surpassed my wildest dreams!" They are asked to deliver it to the group three times in succession. The first with no gestures accompanying it, the second time with an emphatic gesture accompanying it, and the third time with a great big, over-the-top, Academy Award winning gesture. Can you guess what happens? As the gestures get bigger, the voice and volume follow! Inflating your hand gestures, and thereby your vocal delivery, is a simple way to enlarge your whole presence. You are now more noticeable, more memorable!

Don't do dumb things with your body that say "I'm nervous, or uncomfortable, or weird".

You know what these things are:

- fidget, twitch or scratch
- play with your hair
- fluttery hand movements
- slouch
- head down
- avoid eye contact
- touch your face
- sit low in your chair or lean back
- giggle
- continuously push your glasses onto your nose
- swing your leg
- vibrate your foot
- use um, er, or other fillers
- hold your head up by cupping your chin in your hand
- sniff

We all have some of these ungainly habits to watch out for. What are yours?

_____

_____

_____

3. The Handshake

We can all describe the bad handshakes we've gotten; limp, sweaty, bone-crushing, hesitant, or too familiar. The handshake is one of the very first things that someone experiences of you, it's absolutely worth spending some time making it work for you. You want to master a great handshake: firm (but not crushing) grip; two or three solid pumps, eye contact, and a smile.

Whenever you meet a new person, introduce yourself and extend your hand for a good firm handshake. This is a risk-free way of initiating rather than responding.

4. Find Something In Common

Think of people who upon first meeting, you instantly liked, felt comfortable with, and wanted to spend more time with. Why do think this was so? More than likely it's because the two of you found something in common. An interest, a home town, an age bracket, an opinion. I met my friend Carrie a number of years back in a hockey arena, looking for the right place to be for our sons' team tryouts. There we both were; two 35+, harried, blonde, working, single hockey moms in the wrong dressing room. Instant connection!

Do what you can to discover any clues about another person which might provide a common link between you. For example:

> "You have an interesting accent, sounds like you may have a European background? My family is originally from Germany".

> "Hey, did you ever take swimming lessons as a kid?"

> "I see you're reading Jim Collins' latest book. I just finished it too. What do you think of it?"

> "I see you are reading a horticultural magazine. Do you love to garden as I do?"

> "I can see by your jacket that there is a hockey involvement in your family. Are you a hockey parent as I am?"

> "I see by the family portrait on your desk that you have three lovely daughters. I have daughters too. It's an interesting adventure, isn't it?"

5. Show Genuine Interest

"People don't care how much you know until they know how much you care ... about them." John Maxwell

The authors of *First Impressions; What You Don't Know About How Others See You* tell us this: "There are few hard and fast rules for making a positive first impression, but here's one: You will come across more positively if you show genuine interest in people you meet for the first time." Why? Because people are highly tuned in to others' interest in them. They feel it when it's there, and they feel it even more when it's missing.

Think of some of the most painful, boring interactions you've had. The ones where your partner's conversation was exclusively focussed on themselves, they asked no questions of you, they showed not a scrap of interest in you. Memorable exchanges indeed, but for all the wrong reasons!

Active Listening
As an introvert, we do tend to be thought of as good listeners. This may or may not be true. So the trick to this strategy is that it is genuine. Time to fess up. Have you been guilty of standing there nodding your head, appearing to be listening but all the while inwardly rolling your eyes or formulating an escape strategy?

Active listening is a great way to show genuine interest. It involves focussing all your attention on the speaker, avoiding external or internal distractions, maintaining eye contact, asking probing questions, and it can mean paraphrasing the speaker's words, to show we seek clarity and understanding.

Showing interest is also noticing something about them and commenting on it, being complementary, and being respectful of an opinion even when you don't share it.

The more you show a genuine interest in someone, the more they will notice you, remember you, and want to spend time with you. It's because they feel good in your presence!

6. What Your Words Are Saying About You!

I do a lot of coaching with clients in the area of use of language. Many people are quite unaware of the messages that their choice of words impart. Words are very powerful!

Some people's speech is full of phrases which take away their personal power. Here are some examples of how to make a stronger impression just by choosing different words:

Instead of saying...	...Try this instead
I don't really know	Well, I'm not too sure about that, but here's something I do know...
I think that...	I'm sure you'll find that...

Thank you for giving me your time today…	It's been a great pleasure to speak with you today, thank you!.
I really enjoyed it.	It was incredible/fabulous/awesome/the best ever/truly awe-inspiring!
Maybe you could…	What I'd like you to do now is…
Research will be presented by Jean at the conference. (Passive voice)	Jean will present the research at the conference. (Active voice)
I don't see why not.	This will be no problem at all!
The only thing I can do is…	Here is what I suggest we do…
Yah, but…	Yes, and…
I'll try…	I will…

Got any of your own favourites? I'd love to hear from you and will include them in a **Splash** workshop or talk!

_____

_____

_____

If you believe in this sort of thing as I do, check out some resources on neuro-linguistic programming (NLP). Powerful stuff! The easy to digest book, *Neuro-Linguistic Programming for Dummies* by Romilla Ready and Kate Burton is a great foundation.

My Action Plan
By now you know what to do next. Right. Review your thoughts and notes from the 6 techniques above, and jot them down on the following worksheets. Once again, don't worry about filling in every square, just make a note of the strategies that you feel will make the biggest difference for you.

"Do Your Best Dive First" Making Memorable First Impressions	This area definitely needs fine tuning. Some ideas that could work for me are… Specifically, with whom? In which situations?
Your Take on The Lake (how's your attitude?)	
Stories Your Body is Telling (how's your body language?)	
The Handshake	
Find Something in Common	
Show Genuine Interest	
What Your Words Are Saying About You (are you giving up your power?)	

Now, looking at each great idea, think about which would be relatively painless, and changes that you can make starting right now.

_____

_____

_____

_____

Consider which strategies will be a little tougher. What is challenging about these for you, and what can you do to help yourself make them happen?

_____

_____

_____

_____

As Cheryl, a successful sales support specialist tells us wisely "It doesn't have to be a big deal. I just trained myself to smile, introduce myself, and extend my hand to shake. I tell a story, and listen to theirs."

The real art of conversation is not only to say the right thing in the right place, but also to leave unsaid the wrong thing at the tempting moment.

Splash Strategy 4 - Bring A Life Preserver

"Energy and persistence alter all things." Benjamin Franklin

This chapter is all about energy. The big idea is for you to be in control (or at least more in control) over where and how you spend your energy. Versus allowing the people and circumstances around you to dictate. Sound good?

So what follows are strategies to help you:
- make deliberate choices about where and how you'll invest your energy,
- turn it up when you need to, and
- re-energize when you're out of steam.

What Do Introverts Look Like When Their Energy Pool is Drained?

The following are taken from the input of the real-life introverts who participated in our splash workshops and surveys regarding what it's like when their energy is depleted:

- Frustrated, cranky
- Down, depressed
- Hopeless (when I can't escape)
- Shun the company of others, even though I really like/love them
- Unable to think clearly
- Unable to make decisions
- Can't find my words.
- Avoid eye contact at all cost
- Feel overwhelmed
- Get very annoyed when someone tries to "perk me up"
- Useless
- Short-tempered, snappy
- Feel like I'm "not myself"

EXERCISE #1

What is it like for you when your energy is spent?

_____

_____

_____

_____

The Difference Between Managing Your Energy and "Copping Out"

Just to be clear folks, this is not about coddling, making excuses or devising escape strategies (well maybe just a few.) It's about being more purposefully in control of where and how you invest your precious energy.

So let's start with taking a closer look at what is happening for you right now in your energy pool. Take some down time and think about the following questions:

EXERCISE #2

When Do I Float? What Makes Me Sink?

At what time of day do I have the most energy?

_____

At what time of day is it best for me to exercise?

_____

At what time of day is it best for me to interact with people?

_____

How about the really chatty ones?

_____

What kinds of activities or situations energize me?

_____

What kinds of activities or situations do I avoid when I'm out of energy?

_____

What drains my energy the most?

_____

What am I like when I'm pooped?

_____

What's it like when I'm at the top of my energy game?

_____

So...

What did you learn from that exercise? Notice any trends? Any surprises? Any hot buttons? Any truths?

_____

_____

_____

_____

Expectations and Realities

What are the big energy challenges for you? Do you believe you are "required" to spend energy in ways you'd rather not because of pressure (either real or perceived) from family members, your position, your job, your partner, your boss, your spouse?

What about timing? Do you have the least energy in the morning, but are required to expend it then because of family or professional activities? Are you totally pooped at the end of the day, and then need to keep going because of personal, family or professional obligations?

EXERCISE **#3**
Take a Ride on the Magic Wave.

If you could rearrange how and when you expend your energy, what would your day look like? What would you be doing differently? What would others be doing differently? What would your work look like? What would the weekend look like? Think big, as if anything is possible. This exercise is about visualization, so you may want to include going to a quiet place, giving yourself plenty of time, closing your eyes, a glass of good red wine...

_____

_____

_____

_____

_____

_____

Making Your Fantasy a Reality

Now we're clearer on what the ideal state would be. You could be saying to yourself, "As if THAT could ever happen. It's just not my reality." I will challenge you now to put that attitude aside. Instead, open up to the possibility that there are things you can take control of, that will get you a whole lot closer to that ideal state than you are now. Sound worth it? Good.

We'll spend the rest of this chapter looking at some specific strategies to move you closer to your fantasy world, as far as being in control of how, when and where you invest your energy. As you review them, make some notes on the ones that appeal to you. Then we'll revisit your goals, and decide on which strategies you will try on for size.

1. Be Selective and Proactive

"In order to stay in control and out of trouble, you should always be in charge of your own transportation, your own birth control, and your own alarm clock."
                                                                                    Carole Cameron

This is about being at the helm of your energy ship. It's about giving yourself permission to do more of what works for you, and less of what doesn't. Of course it involves knowing yourself pretty well, and hopefully earlier on in the chapter we've helped you bring your energy preferences into focus a little better.

Be clear about how many extra-curricular activities you can handle in a week. Social engagements, hockey parties, book club, volleyball, choir practice, and the like. As they say at the casinos "know your limit and play within it." Raj has this down to a tee. He tells us "I know that my limit for evenings out with activities is 2-3 per week. This includes the weekend. (It also allows for unavoidable things that pop up and must be attended to.) So if I have a hot date lined up for the weekend, I only do one other extra-curricular thing during the week. I just don't sign up for everything that catches my fancy, and I'm getting pretty good at just saying no."

This takes some planning for sure, but then you are in control. You can plan your week. If you are participating in a high-energy day at work, don't plan a social activity, or one that requires more energy for that particular evening. Or, more pro-actively put, plan a quiet, recharging activity for that evening. True, it's not always possible, but if you do it when you can, you are further down the road to your ideal state.

When you plan out your week, look at each day and schedule in some down time. A busy mom I know schedules a nap in for everyday for 30 minutes, just before the kids get home from school. She has trained the folks in her life that she is not available at this particular time each day, so for the most part, they don't call or stop by.

Marc, a successful corporate financial director blocks off time each day for down time. He plugs it all into his electronic calendar on Sunday night, or a few weeks in advance. Other events and meetings are scheduled around it. During this oasis time he shuts his door, and does important thinking, strategizing, or writing. The time is booked off as busy on his calendar for all to see so they work around it. It takes discipline to do it, and to not give it away when things get busy, but it keeps him sane, unfrazzled and better prepared to be energized for everything else.

There are lots of different reasons why we join things, say yes to requests, meet with our friends, attend meetings, and volunteer for things. Often because we want to be involved in an activity that we enjoy. Sometimes because we feel obligated. Take a look at all your extra-curricular activities. Are there any that you are just doing because you feel obligated? Are there any that you keep doing only because you've been doing them for years? Are there some that energize you just thinking about them? Are there any activities you've been thinking that you'd really enjoy, but feel you can't fit them in along with everything else?

We suggest not just saying no, but prioritizing. Identify the activities that are not enjoyable any more, not essential, you really detest, or that just plain suck the energy out of you. Then eliminate them. Don't re-join the board next year. Don't organize the school fund raiser just because you've done it for the past 4 years. Let someone else take over. Say no to the wild party at the home of friends who you really don't enjoy or respect anymore. Enjoy the freedom to fill these spaces with energizing activities, be they restful, or more fulfilling for you. Your energy pool is finite and precious! Don't waste it.

No, No, No!

"It's been fun to run the hockey pool for the last 8 years, and now it's time for someone else to have the pleasure. This will be my last year."

"I'm sorry we have plans for that evening. But please think of us next time."

"I won't be able to collect door to door this year but I would like to give a donation."

"I won't be able to attend the whole event, would it be alright to stop in for an hour?"

"You've done such wonderful work with the choir, and I'm sorry I won't be able to take on the leadership at this time. Thank you so much for thinking of me, I'm flattered."

"Let me check my schedule and I'll let you know."

Think about all the extra-curricular activities you are involved in regularly, and those which come up every so often. Which would you be willing to eliminate?

_____

_____

_____

_____

Add, Keep, or Toss

This includes making decisions about the people you choose to spend your time with too. Give some thought to the people in your life that you spend time with. There are ones who build you up and energize you. With them you feel alive, natural, comfortable and fabulous. They bring out the best in you, and you add to their lives too. Let's call this the *A List*.

The *B List* contains the ones who you need to spend time with because of the realities and circumstances in your life; you don't usually get to pick your co-workers or your family.

And then there's the *C List*. Who's on it? The people in your life who simply drain you. Suck the life-blood out of you. You cringe when you see their name on the call display. You really don't enjoy spending time with them, but you do because you feel you have to or you should. Maybe an old friend you've outgrown, maybe someone with too many troubles, maybe someone who just doesn't know when to stop talking. Maybe someone so negative or miserable or mean that after even a short time with them you come away feeling down, or even trampled on.

Think of the people in your life. Who's on which list?

A List:

_____

_____

_____

B List:

_____

_____

_____

C List:

_____

_____

_____

Yes of course you know what comes next. Think about the folks on your *C List.* Which would you be willing to eliminate (or at least reduce) from your life?

_____

_____

_____

For some this is a very tough thing to consider doing. For others, you may do this naturally anyway. How do you manage *C Listers* out of your life? In one way or another you just say no. You are busy when they ask you to come over or go out, you have a great reason to cut the call short when they phone, you stop including them in group events. You act in a way that doesn't allow them to suck you dry, and they will go away. For example...

I had a friend who, over the years, had a series of relationships with men that had ended badly. She was not willing to take accountability for her own part in those relationships, and over the years she became a bitter, self-pitying man-hater. She also blamed everyone else she could for her sad state; her job, her boss, her mother, etc. (Astoundingly, she also couldn't figure out why she couldn't find a good man!) Spending time with her was no longer enjoyable or energizing. My feedback or advice was not welcome nor heeded, although she continued to seek out contact with me. I decided that I needed to manage her out of my life. I stopped being a sympathetic ear, and started to talk about only positive things and possibilities. I did not get sucked into commiserating in the "men are pigs" discussion. I shared with her only the happiest and most fulfilling experiences in my relationships. Can you guess what eventually happened? She disappeared and found another partner for her pity-party.

Just a final note about saying NO
This strategy comes with a warning. It is only to be used by mature, evolved,

grown-up introverts. It is not, I repeat <u>not</u> to be used as an excuse or cop out.

Say no to conserve your energy in order to spend it on the things you really want to. Say no if you just will not have the energy to be at your best. Don't say no because you'd just rather not go out of your way, or you want to escape. Remember, you are creating your life the way you want it to be.

Rest before you get pooped
Plan to charge up before a high energy event, that way you'll be in high gear and be at your best. Also, you won't have the same kind of crash to deal with afterwards. If you know you are going to a party on Saturday night, spend the day in quieter activities on your own. Gardening, reading, walking, working out, cooking, watching a movie, whatever your favourites are.

Create a smaller pond
Many introverts feel overwhelmed initially when they arrive at a party or large business function. Generally they feel more comfortable in smaller groups, and with people they know. John tells us what he does at a larger function to create a smaller, more intimate environment for himself. "When I walk into a large group of people, I scan the room for anyone I know. I feel ok approaching them and entering into a conversation. But you don't want to monopolize anyone for the whole night. I also don't necessarily want to talk to as many people as possible, just a selective few who I would enjoy. Sometimes I'll walk around looking at the art, or something. I try not too look too deep in thought, or unapproachable, and usually, someone will approach me with a little conversation starter. I welcome their company. Sometimes I'll find a place a little off to the side. I may be there by myself, or I may join someone else who has already found it. We can have a lovely conversation, and then other folks may join us, and come and go. It's kind of a mini-party within a party."

2. Ask for What You Want

"We can only dream that someday, when our condition is more widely understood, when perhaps an Introverts' Rights movement has blossomed and borne fruit, it will not be impolite to say I'm an introvert. You are a wonderful person and I like you. But now please shush." Jonathan Raunch

In my opinion, too much of what is written for introverts has themes like "survival strategies", or "managing in an extroverted world". What is often missing is advice on how to "make things more the way you'd like them". Once again, about being more in control. Here's an example: Carole-Anne is a lovely, very intelligent, academically oriented, imaginative introvert. She has a strong preference that social interaction be one-on-one, wherein there is the opportunity for deeper conversation and exploration of ideas. So, often when she's invited to join a friend at a big party or gathering, she'll say something like "thank you for asking me, and I would really like to spend time with you. Can we arrange a date when we can meet one-on-one?" Brilliant! Ask for what you want.

When planning to go to a party or function, tell the host beforehand that you will need to leave at X o'clock. That way you'll know you only have to be charming and adorable for a few hours, and then you're done. If you end up having a great time, you can always tell your host you've made arrangements that will allow you to stay longer. Of course, if you have a partner, you'll need to negotiate this in advance. A few couples I know have an understanding that it's ok for one partner to leave the party and one to stay.

At the beginning of a phone call which has the potential to go on longer than you'd like, tell your caller that you have a conference call or an appointment in 20 minutes. (It isn't necessarily dishonest; you may have an appointment with your washing machine!) This allows you to end the call when you want to, and also helps to ensure that your caller has covered the important stuff within the time frame.

Ask for what you want in social or group conversations:

> "Thanks for such a nice chat. I need to have a quick word with my boss"
> "I'm on my way now, but I'd love to connect with you again sometime. Here's my card, may I call you?"
> "Excuse me, I need to check in on the dog-sitter"
> "Well I'm going to go now and check out what's happening at the food table!"
> "I must leave you now, I promised my colleague I'd buy him a drink tonight"
> "I've enjoyed our chat, I'm going to get another drink, maybe we can talk some more later."

Ask for what you want at work and at home:

Explain your introverted preferences to you boss, your colleagues, your family and friends so you are not misunderstood. Tell your work colleagues that, although it may appear that you are not participating in a meeting, you are actually processing and thinking, and would appreciate the opportunity to comment or add to the discussion after the fact. Tell them that your most brilliant moments come after a chance to reflect, and that they can often expect an email or a one-on-one meeting later. Tell your friends that although you love them dearly, you do not always have the energy it takes to enjoy them fully, and would sometimes prefer a short chat on the phone to a long visit. Tell your extraverted friend that you can visit with him for two days while you're in town, but not four as he suggested.

If possible, swap family duties to suit the times of day when you have the most energy. For example, if you really prefer to start your day quietly, see if you can arrange for your partner to drop the kids at day-care, allowing you some time in the silent house before heading out, then your job is the pick-up. If your energy is high in the morning and wanes as the day goes on, be in charge of breakfast, bed-making, and lunches while your partner is on duty for dinner.

Shirley tells a great story about a fabulous trip she took to Britain with three extraverted friends, and what she learned from it:

> "As it turned out, most of the clothes I had packed went home with me un-worn. I assumed that we would, as I usually do, return to the hotel each day to unwind and dress for dinner. Well, there was no returning to the hotel! We left each morning at 9am, walked for six to eight hours a day, go go go from one thing to the next, and there was no thinking about what we'd do, we just "did" whatever was there at the time, wherever we happened to end up! We'd have a nice dinner, and then look for more places to go and things to see! It was non-stop! In the galleries, palaces, or museums I escaped into corners to concentrate on art or monuments, or things relating to the books I've read. I felt panicky in the crowds in places like Piccadilly Circus (which we retuned to 3 times because the extraverts loved it there). I felt physically uncomfortable there, where we were pushed and bumped and warned to look out for pickpockets. I had a great time, saw everything tourists should see, shared lots of laughter, and I'm truly happy that I went. But as an introvert, I don't feel like I had a "vacation".

Shirley learned some great lessons for all of us when planning a trip or vacation with family and friends: When in the planning phase, make your request for pockets of down time clearly known. Make an agreement that everyone doesn't have to do everything, and it's ok to opt out of an activity or tour. Asking for what you want up front can head off misunderstandings, exhaustion, crabbiness, or other things which can lessen the enjoyment of a great vacation.

3. Manage Technology, Don't Let it Manage You

I used to cringe when my phone rang, and curse the emails that kept popping up, nagging for my attention. I used to swear that I'd never get a Blackberry because I wanted to be the one in control of my time and how I spend it. I had a rather limited view of what technology can do for me, I just needed to learn how to manage it better. A couple of time management courses later, coupled with some discipline, and I've developed new habits which put me in the driver's seat. I'll share these with you, along with some great tips from other splashy introverts:

Pick a couple of windows in the day when it makes sense for you to respond to voicemails and emails. I like to deal with them mid-morning, mid afternoon, and at the end of the day. This way I can avoid the aggravated feeling of being interrupted (how dare they!) and get myself revved up to respond energetically. As much as possible, I let people know that I generally respond to email and voice mails in those time periods.

Pick your times, then avoid the urge to peek at your emails unless you are expecting an important message. Screen your phone calls using call display, and only answer those which are critical. Let the rest go to voice mail. Use your voice mail greeting to maximum advantage. Steve Prentice, author of Cool – Time and the Two-Pound Bucket suggests something like this:

"You've reached Chris Roberts of XYZ Company for Tuesday the 16th. I will be in a meeting this morning and will be returning calls between 11:00 and noon, and again between 2:30 and 3:30. Please leave a detailed message and I will return your call. If this message is urgent, please press 0 to reach my assistant (or give your cell phone number). Thanks for calling, and have a great day!"

I realize this strategy will not work for everyone, you may have a job such as in service, or support, which requires you to answer the phone when it rings. Even so, try at home to check in only so often.

4. Ramping it Up When You Need To

"Every introvert is an actor." Dustin Hoffman

I like to keep fit by running. I'm not really competitive, but every so often I'll get some friends together and we'll enter a race. The excitement and energy level at the race event site is so amazing! Those of you who've stood at the finish line as runners are coming in have seen many of them crank up a burst of speed and sprint through the finish line. Where does that energy burst come from? It comes from the runner's preparation for the event, and from the thrill of the event. A good runner trains for weeks, and comes prepared to do his or her very best. This strategy is about introverts deliberately being prepared and willing to pull it out of the bag when it's important to. Once again, about acting purposefully because you know the results are worth it.

Take On A Persona
Many introverts tell us about *flipping the switch*, or *psyching myself up*. They are referring to deliberately taking on another persona which is the most effective for the situation at hand.

Michael shares with us: "When I need to, I switch on my "extravert persona" and away I go. It's almost like firing turbo jets to get through a situation. (Of course turbo jets require a lot of refuelling afterwards)"

The Power of the Marker
I use this phrase as a metaphor for the power of the role. What I mean is that certain roles, or levels of seniority, or positions afford us the opportunity to act and appear more out there, more confident, bigger, faster, more energized. In my role as a facilitator, I am most effective in the classroom when I'm highly energized and larger than life. I need to be rested and revved up for it and crash after it, but it's what makes for an enjoyable, sustainable, and memorable learning experience. When I have the *marker in my hand*, I can transform myself from a quiet, thoughtful, solitary training developer into a dynamic facilitator. Because that's what the role requires.

At work as a sales manager, Pat is energetic, articulate and swift to action. His role calls for it, and he rises to the occasion when with customers and his sales staff. "(this kind of behaviour) is an expectation for excellent performance and results in this role" he says.

The Power of the Mask
Do you remember going to a costume party? Maybe for a themed party like on Oscar night, where you'd come dressed as your favourite actor, perhaps Clarke Gable or Marilyn Monroe. Or as a youngster putting on your Hallowe'en costume and walking door to door in the dark, calling "Trick or Treat" to your neighbours. Do you remember what a kick it was when your best friend's mom didn't recognize you? What a thrill anonymity can bring! And what freedom! And what a great opportunity to practice some new behaviours. Why not attend an event where you are a complete stranger, and try on some *Splash* strategies. If they work for you, great! If they don't go quite as planned, no worries, nobody knows you anyway. Nor did they notice what you were doing. Anonymity is as much a mask as any one of those plastic super-hero or princess ones you wore as a kid. And you can breathe through the nose holes much better.

"Acting As If"
"Acting as if" is a very powerful tool to help you get from where you are to where you wish to be. The idea has been around a while, perhaps you've heard about it at a motivational seminar, or on a developmental tape, or read about it. It's related to visualization, which athletes and other top-performers use.

"Acting as if" means you pretend for the moment, or the evening, that you actually possess the quality that you wish to acquire. For example, you decide that at tonight's networking event, you are going to "act as if" you are charming and outgoing. You determine what the specific behaviours of a charming and outgoing person are, and then you do your best to behave that way. Maybe you go for being complementary, initiating conversations, making solid eye contact and displaying good energy. The strategy gives you permission and an opportunity to try on new behaviour and see what happens. The idea is that if you practice long enough, the acting is no longer acting, but rather doing what comes more naturally.

Think what it would be like to "act as if" in the examples below. What would you be doing? What would you be saying?

- Acting as if you are brave.
- Acting as if you aren't shy
- Acting as if you are attractive.
- Acting as if you are happy.
- Acting as if you are a powerful presenter.
- Acting as if you have a positive attitude.

Here's another spin on this tool:

- If I were a world famous author, what would I be doing/saying now?
- If I were a top sales person, what would I be doing/saying now?
- If I were a charming conversationalist, what would I be doing/saying now?
- If I were confident, what would I be doing/saying now?

Think of an opportunity to try on new behaviour by coaching yourself this way and see what happens.

Using Language For Energy
This is a simple way to up your energy; on the inside and the outside! Use high energy words like "fabulous!", "incredible", "stunning", "passionate" "excited", "amazing!", "sounds great!" instead of "ok", "fine", "nice", and "all right".

Pay attention to the emotional tone of your speech, and notch it up. You've probably come across the tip at customer service seminars about "putting a smile in your voice". The idea is to remember to smile first, and then answer the telephone, the smile will come through in your voice. Does it actually work? Of course it works!!

Using Humour
A couple of great suggestions came from our *Splash* workshop participants regarding humour, and its relationship to energy.

Ajay shared with us; "Even if I'm not "the life of the party", I can still tell a pretty good joke. I have found that once people see I have a good sense of humour, they find me more likeable and approachable. Then, once engaged with someone, I can find more energy to work with."

Donna, a marketing manager says "I'm a pretty intense person. Sometimes I just find I'm taking everything far too seriously. It's actually comical at times, when you think about it. Like as if what happens in the office supplies market is going to change the world. I saw a great training video once, and I'll always remember this part of it. They said "Remember Rule #6" Rule #6 is "don't take yourself so $%^& seriously." When I do remember this, I almost instantly lighten up, brighten up, and can find it a little easier to find the energy I need at the moment."

5. Float with the Extraverts for a While (but just a little while…)

I love my extraverted friends. I am amused, entertained, enthralled and energized by them. As a matter of fact, my life would be extra-ordinarily different were it not for a few lucky encounters with a few special extraverts.

In elementary school, I was identified as a candidate for an "advanced" learning experience, a new thing to our city at the time. So, at the age of 10, I lined up every morning with a few others from my home school, and waited for the yellow school bus to come. For five years, I travelled daily on that bus, and went to school with students who lived in all different parts of the city. I loved my school and had lots of friends, but my old neighbourhood friendships dropped off. When it came time to go to high school back in the neighbourhood, I knew no one. I was terrified! I figured everyone else would know everyone else already. How would I meet people and fit in? I knew that being chatty and meeting new people was not my forté. My older brother reluctantly agreed to walk with me to school that first day. As we three hundred or so grade niners sat in the auditorium, waiting for our names to be called by our new homeroom teacher, one of the girls I had been friends with in pre-bus days came over to say hello. Debbie is friendly, outgoing, totally social and completely likeable, and needless to say, extraverted. Because of her, and through her, I was able to meet new people, go to dances, get invited to parties, and have an absolutely fabulous time in high school. Debbie was also gracious enough to share her extensive network of friends with me, in which I discovered another soulmate and life-long friend, Lyn. I always wonder what those high school days (and the rest of my life) would have been like if she hadn't initiated that contact.

It's great to tap into that extraverted energy source! I love to work with the high energy folks, to brainstorm, to debate, to discuss. I need extraverts in my workshops to liven things up! In her best-selling book, *The Introvert Advantage*, Marti Olsen Laney coins the phrase "catching confidence". When we rise to the occasion with the extroverted gang, it's like "catching energy". Of course the time spent with them needs to be managed and balanced and limited, but it's worth it! And remember, it's about getting energized, not exhausted!
Lisa offered this fabulous suggestion for riding on the wave of an extravert's energy in order to make the most of those dreaded networking events: "Try connecting with an extravert when going to a networking event. Going two-by-two is often more fun anyway, and since the extravert can "work the room" with ease, they can also introduce their friend the introvert. It's a good buddy system, which can produce win-win results."

6. Refresh With the Introverts

"There was a pause, just long enough for an angel to pass, flying slowly"
     Ronald Firbank, on how introverts tend to pause to think before they speak.

One way to re-energize is to deliberately make time to hang out with your introverted friends. Meet them to talk, discuss a book, chat about work, go for a workout, or for dinner and drinks. It's a great way to meet social, intellectual or physical fitness needs, and to not get annoyed or exhausted while doing it!

I have a group of 4 friends, all introverted. We meet for drinks and dinner as often as our schedules allow, and we all bask in the comfort and calmness of our introverted preference. No interrupting to get a point across or to get a word in edgewise. Just a lovely, gentle, rhythmic exchange of ideas and experiences. Gotta love it. I invariably come home relaxed and refreshed. Who is in your introverted network?

7. Eat, Drink, Sleep, and Exercise.

A fit, healthy body is an energetic being.

Eat
Support your energy pool with good health and wellness habits. Think back to a time when you were trying to drop a few pounds. You cut out the carbs, and tried to eat less of everything else. Do you remember how you felt in the energy department? Sluggish? No surprise. Low-carbohydrate, low calorie diets deplete energy. Fad and extreme dieting causes your metabolism to go into hibernation, preparing your body for the scant quantities of food you're giving it. You need your metabolism high to burn fat and give you physical energy. To maintain energy you need to nourish your body with high quality, real food. Especially lean protein and complex carbohydrates. I'm not a nutritionist by any means, but I've learned a lot from reading and from my personal trainer. I suggest getting educated about nutrition, and making some healthy choices.

Here are some very general guidelines to eating for health and energy:

- Avoid the sugary, greasy, and processed stuff like pop, cookies, donuts, French fries, fast food, packaged food.
- Avoid simple carbs like potatoes, white rice, white pasta, white rice.
- Eat complex carbs (this is where our body gets the energy) like whole grains, fresh fruit and vegetables, beans, oatmeal.

- Eat only healthy fats like olive oil, flaxseed oil, sunflower seeds, almonds, avocado.
- Eat lean protein like chicken breast, white fish, salmon, tuna, egg whites, turkey.
- Avoid high fat meats like marbled red meat, ground beef, bacon, processed deli meats.
- Eat more, smaller meals each day.
- Eat breakfast. Definitely eat breakfast.

Drink

Water, that is. We've all heard it a million times. Drink six to eight glasses of water a day. Without enough water, our bodies become dehydrated. Symptoms, among many others, are fatigue, lethargy, irritability, lack of mental clarity, headache. Not what we're going for. Try this in order to get it all in: drink a half-cup of water every waking hour on the hour.

Sleep

Enough sleep is essential for good health and maximizing energy! Lack of sleep causes your metabolism to slow down. This results in less energy for your day. How much sleep is enough? By now you probably know how much sleep you need to feel rested. Studies show that people who sleep between six and a half to seven and a half hours a night, live the longest. Interesting. The point is, make it a priority to deliberately get enough sleep.

Exercise

Working out regularly elevates the endorphins which makes us feel more lively and energetic. Some people will say "I'm too tired to exercise." Well it might be how you feel, but the truth is that exercising will increase your energy level and your endurance level. The more consistent you are with your visits to the health club, or to the pavement, or with your treadmill in the basement, the more stable your level of energy will be during the rest of your day.

Get some guidance to create a workout regime including both cardiovascular and weight training. A minimum of three to five times per week.

When is the best time to work out? Ideally, the time of day you have the most energy is the best time to work out. If this works with your lifestyle, great! If not, do it when you can. However you go about it is up to you but working out and staying active will give you more energy and keep your energy levels higher throughout the day either way!

8. Colourful Tips

Remember we talked about the four different varieties of introverts? Do you remember which colour(s) you figured you are? The following strategies for re-energizing and managing energy are examples from "real-life" members of each of the Personality Dimensions colour groups:

Resourceful Orange

- Taking action, but solo. For example, play guitar, play computer games, fix the car
- Take a nap,
- Go for a solitary run or walk,
- Ignore emails and voicemails,
- Refrain from talking with anyone,
- Driving the car fast,
- Working out,
- Listening to music,
- Grabbing a relaxing moment "on the go". Sneak in a nap, or a walk,
- Trying out new recipes,
- Going to a bike, or snowmobile shop,
- Going for a drive out of town. It's like an escape.

Inquiring Green

- Doing crosswords, Sudoku, or computer scrabble
- Writing something profound,
- Reading something interesting,
- Thinking about a project, and all the different possibilities,
- Ignoring or turning off my Blackberry for at least one hour each day during business hours,
- Going to a book store,
- Googling all those nagging questions I've saved up in my head (what IS bee pollen, anyway?),
- Watching foreign movies with subtitles,
- Figuring out the guitar cords for a tricky riff,
- Challenging needlework,
- Phone? What phone?
- Watching Star Trek re-runs (just kidding)

Authentic Blue

- Doing yoga,
- Writing,
- Journaling,
- Reading a good book, especially one with characters I can connect with
- Dancing,
- Going to an art gallery, theatre or concert,

- Spending time outdoors,
- Retreating to a forest or high desert,
- Going for a long quiet walk which provides time to daydream,
- Tuning out the world,
- Blogging about the causes I'm interested in,
- Going golfing,
- Antiquing,
- Listening to classical music.

Organized Gold

- Sitting quietly and reading for 15 or 20 minutes before leaving for work,
- Turning off the tv and radio,
- Reading quietly,
- Planning and preparing meals for the whole week,
- Taking a break by watching a favourite television show from my PVR
- Finishing a project,
- Planning a family vacation,
- Balance my cheque book.
- Scrapbooking
- Working out on my lunch hour,
- Getting organized (or reorganized) is totally energizing.
- Shopping for Christmas gifts, birthday presents and cards well ahead of time.

My Action Plan

Now what? Review your thoughts and notes from the 8 techniques above, and jot down the ones you think you'd like to try on for size.

"Bring a Life Preserver" Managing Energy	Some ideas that I'd like to try out are… Specifically with whom, in which situations?
Be Selective and Proactive	
Ask For What You Want	
Manage Technology vs it Managing You	
Zipping it Up When You Need To	
Float with the Extraverts for a While	
Refresh with the Introverts	
Eat, Drink, Sleep and Exercise	
Colourful Tips	

Now, looking at each great idea, think about which ones would be relatively painless, and which ones that you can start doing right now.

_____

_____

_____

_____

Now consider which strategies could be a little tougher. What is challenging about these for you, and what could you do to support yourself to do them?

_____

_____

_____

_____

Splash Strategy 5 - Find a New Pond

You can never discover new oceans unless you are prepared to lose site of the shore.

This chapter is about making the big changes in your life. These could include things like a new job, a new career, the beginning of a new relationship or the end of an existing one. Perhaps moving to a new home or city or country. Maybe deciding to lose 60 pounds or to train for a marathon.

Earlier we talked of the 3 choices we have when we are in a situation with which we are not completely satisfied:

1. grin and bear it,
2. improve it, or
3. change it completely.

I suppose this chapter adds a fourth choice to the list; "blow it out of the water."

The big changes are hard! They are often overwhelming, scary and involve real risks. You can certainly enhance your life significantly by embracing the *Splash* strategies we've talked about so far. Perhaps you already have! This chapter builds on those. You'll find more supportive tools and attitudes which can help you make the really big changes you want, once the time is right.

Sometimes tweaking the way things are isn't quite enough. Sometimes, in order to get to where you really want to be, you need to take a flying leap off the high diving board.

It would be foolish and irresponsible to suggest that anyone make a huge change in their life (quit your job, start a business, buy real estate, leave your spouse, have a child, shun your sister) just for the thrill of it although for many, big changes can be quite exhilarating and tempting. We make these important choices only if it's what the doctor orders. (Remember, you are the doctor.) If we're wise, we take life-changing action only after sufficient consideration and thought.

Here's how it went for me: I spent the first half of my career working for others; being employed in positions with companies, including spending 10 plus years in the seriously corporate arena. The corporate experience was extremely valuable, I learned a ton, met amazing people, made valuable contacts, was trained and mentored by the best in the industry, and was influenced in life-changing ways by a few incredible people. However, I've always been a bit of a non-conformist; not necessarily buying into all the processes and procedures that I was to uphold and teach, or sometimes giggling at things that others didn't find funny.

After a while, I began to feel a little like I was just playing a game, and was not completely satisfied or committed to my work. I just couldn't take training workshops with messages like "think outside the box" or "paradigm shifts" all that seriously. (I suppose after a while they couldn't take me all that seriously either!).

I had been dreaming for years of working independently as a consultant, but the time never seemed right, and the risk seemed too great. Eventually, the right time did appear, thanks to a prickly no-win situation with a new boss. So, before getting fired, I decided it was time to fly on my own. I proposed a contract for a few days per week of consulting work with my soon-to-be-former employer for one year. This would take quite a bit of the risk out of the venture, and allow me some space to build the rest of my business. Well what do you know, they agreed! (Talk about the power of asking for what you want!)

Essentially, what once "fit" didn't anymore. The new reality I created fit me perfectly. Working from an office in my home, primarily in solitude, but with enough client and colleague contact to keep me from going stir-crazy or losing creativity. Having a ton of independence and flexibility, (that means things like finishing up a proposal or training design in the morning, and going to the spa in the afternoon). Living and working the way that embraces my core needs for independence, creativity and income.

When I decided to start my own business, the reasons were simple. I wanted to:

- Do more of the things I like
- Do less of the things I don't
- Work with people I really enjoy spending time with

Simple, yes. Easy, no. But just how I like it. It fits! These simple reasons have now evolved into the measures by which I make decisions about assignments. The idea behind creating the life you want is taking a look at what doesn't fit, and considering what would be the perfect fit. Then determining ways to make it happen.

We did a little of this kind of visualization in the previous chapter, when we were talking about being in charge of how you spend your energy. This is the same kind of thing, but bigger!

Get Unstuck
If you keep doing what you've always done you'll keep getting what you've always got.

One important way to know that we need to make a big change in our lives is when we feel "stuck". Michael Bungay Stanier, author of *Get Unstuck and Get*

Going on the Stuff That Matters puts it like this: "stuck is: when you've secretly given up, and you're still in the race", "stuck is: when you're running flat-out and you know you're in the wrong race." You know that you're stuck when what you're currently doing is getting in the way of what you really want to do.

Once again, most introverts don't want to be extroverts. We generally don't necessarily want to be the centre of attention, the CEO, or the things that all those branding books assume we want to be. What we want is to be the best we can be, to develop and use our talents, to show the world our best stuff. To put into and get out of life what makes us happy and fulfilled.

Are You Swimming To Or Swimming Away From?
Luckily for me, as I was eagerly climbing up the ladder to the high diving board in order to jump off and embark on some monumental changes in my life, a bright and thoughtful colleague had the wisdom to advise me "just be sure you're running <u>to</u> something, rather than running <u>away from</u> something". A profound consideration, and a cause for meaningful reflection. Was I running away from a nasty boss or an unpleasant situation? Was it easier for me to change or leave, rather than to deal with the issues at hand?

As you make the big decisions in your life, be sure to check in on your intentions. Sometimes, depending on your "colour", or temperament, or history, it's easier to take a left hand turn than to stick with the situation and fix it. Sometimes, making that big break is the only way out. Just be sure to think on this one, but don't use it as an excuse.

Another Long Look In The Reflection Pool

Exercise #1
Start by reviewing your notes from page 23 where you took an inventory of what was going on in all the areas of your life. Build on that insight with these powerful questions:

Am I "stuck"? (Am I in the wrong race? Have I given up or given in?)

_____

_____

In what?

_____

_____

I have been thinking for quite some time now that I would really like to:

_____

_____

_____

_____

I had a flash of insight a while ago which I can't get out of my head. It was:

_____

_____

I have a "secret" desire to do this:

_____

_____

EXERCISE #2
See if the reflections above have helped you clarify anything you'd really like to be, do or have.

Now consider these questions:

What would a "dream-come-true ending" look like?

_____

_____

On a scale of 1-10, how badly do I want this?

_____

_____

On a scale of 1-10 how truly do I believe it will make life much more the way I want it?

_____

_____

On a scale of 1-10 how hard am I willing to work to make it happen?

_____

_____

What, up to now, has kept me from making this change?

_____

_____

Is this barrier real or perceived?

_____

_____

What are some of the ways I could remove or get around this barrier? (this is the time to get creative!)

_____

_____

_____

_____

Do I have any *cement shoes* which could affect this situation (either the current state or getting to the desired state)?

_____

_____

What do I currently have going for you which supports making this happen?

_____

_____

What or who would help in making this happen?

_____

_____

Who are my greatest fans?

_____

_____

What kind of support can I ask from them?

_____

_____

Who may not be cheering me on from the side of the pool?

_____

_____

What's the best way to deal with them?

_____

_____

What other things could I do which would support my success in making this happen? (Think: learn a new language, get an image consultant, improve public speaking skills, get therapy, lose or gain weight, learn or improve another skill.)

_____

_____

_____

Coaching

Those of you who are familiar with the process of coaching will have recognized that these are typical coaching questions. As you move into action towards all the changes you've decided to make, a life-coach would be ideal. I have seen miraculous transformation in the lives of those I have coached. Coaching helps keep you on track, and keeps you accountable. You can also be your own coach. Self-coaching, I supposed you'd call it.

Coaching is about keeping yourself enthusiastically focussed on your objective, and not letting yourself off the hook. It's about checking in on how you're doing so far, congratulating yourself on it, and moving forward towards the next step. It is keeping yourself moving forward, and not falling back or admitting defeat especially when obstacles show up, or things don't go according to your perfect plan.

From Critic to Coach

Think again about the cement shoes you identified above. Are there things you catch yourself saying that do not help you get where you're going?

See if you can turn that inner voice which is a critic into a coach. How can you turn the messages you feed yourself into helpful, encouraging and empowering ones?

List a few powerful, positive messages that you will use when coaching yourself:

_____

_____

_____

Just Be Fabulous

You may know that you're stuck or spinning, but can't quite find clarity about your next steps. You can't quite visualize the ideal state yet, but you know it's much different from where you are now. I've been there.

A few years back, I was in the midst of a lot of personal transition. My son was about to leave home for university, I had decided I wanted to write a book, I was considering moving from the big city to a smaller town, I wanted to buy a house. I wanted to move my life forward, and I had lots of decisions to make, but the whole thing was just swirling around in my brain. It seemed one decision was dependent on the outcome of another, and that was dependent on some other event which was yet an unknown. I felt paralyzed, because for me, making decisions and taking action is what moves me forward. Thank goodness a friend had the wisdom to say to me "Carole, relax. You don't have to make any of these decisions right now. Just continue to be great at what you do, and save your money. This will equip you for whatever you end up doing." Wow, what a relief! And what freedom! I took his advice, trusted that the answers would appear in their time, (as they did) and was well-prepared to hit the ground running to create the next chapter in my life. I also morphed the advice into my personal motto which pretty much covers and simplifies everything: _"Just Be Fabulous"_.

Have Courage/Be Bold/Be Brave

"Heroes and cowards feel exactly the same way. Heroes react differently, that's all."
Gus D'Amato, boxing trainer

Acting with courage is not about closing your eyes, plugging your nose and jumping right in. It's looking in the water to see where the rocks are, noticing where the current is, and stepping forward with faith in your convictions and your skills. Being brave is not acting without fear. It is not allowing fear to get in the way.

Courage involves trusting yourself. Dr. Benjamin Spock revolutionized parenting with his book, _Baby and Child Care_. It's opening lines: "Trust yourself. You know more than you think you do." Introverts sure know enough about being underestimated to avoid underestimating themselves!

Courage is also being willing to do the work, despite the cost. Being willing to swim through some murky, swamp, stinky waters before getting to the shimmering sea.

"You must do the thing you think you cannot do." Eleanor Roosevelt

Add and Subtract
Which activities, behaviours or habits will I subtract in order to move me faster in the direction I want to go?

_____

_____

_____

Which people in my life will I subtract in order to better support myself getting where I want to go?

_____

_____

_____

What kinds of activities, behaviours and people will I add to my life, in support of getting me what I want?

_____

_____

_____

Turn 40
I say this metaphorically, of course. You may not yet have hit this milestone. But you've gotta believe that as you get a little older, you definitely get wiser in the "get your $#*! together" department. I really wish I could have earlier embraced some of the things that became delightfully true as I matured.

At the risk of being trite (I'm sure you've seen many of these "lists" in the gaggingly profound emails that are forwarded to you each day by well-meaning friends, family and colleagues), here are a few of the lessons in life that I wish I'd known earlier.

What I Learned When I Turned Forty:

- What you think about yourself is far more important than what others think of you.
- It's ok to ask for what you want.
- It's great to say "no".
- It's fabulous to say "yes".
- You don't have to do everything the hard way.
- It's good to be selective. It makes people think you have high standards.
- Don't take yourself so seriously, nobody else does.
- Don't assume malice for what stupidity can explain.
- It's better to be loving than to be right.
- It's ok to believe you're fabulous.
- Dr. Seuss rules.
- You don't have to clean your house before the cleaning lady comes.
- If all else fails, try red wine.

The good news is that you don't have to be over forty to embrace them too!

Swimming The Last Length: Closing Remarks

"We are what we repeatedly do. Excellence then, is not an act, but a habit."
Aristotle

My intention with **Splash** was to share with you what I have learned from swimming along life's stream, and from the brave introverts who have also chosen to create the life experiences that they really want. I sincerely hope that as a result, you've discovered a few pearls that will assist you in getting where you want to go.

Splash is a threefold approach. There's the book, which you have in your hand, a workshop series, and the opportunity for one-on-one coaching.

My story, and yours, is still evolving. I would be thrilled to hear from you about the splashy successes that come your way when you decide to make them happen!

Please feel free to contact me at
carole@makeasplash.ca
www.makeasplash.ca

And will you succeed? Yes indeed, yes indeed! Ninety-eight and three-quarters percent guaranteed! Dr. Seuss

More About Positive Thinking and Getting Your $#*! Together

Feed Your Soul!

I highly recommend reading books and listening to CDs by authors like:

Deepak Chopra
Jim Clemmer
Stephen Covey
Eve Delunas
Wayne Dyer
Ralph Waldo Emerson
Napoleon Hill
William James
Norman Vincent Peale
Eckhart Tolle

There are lots more, send me your favourites!

Backward

Looking back, I should have known Carole Cameron would one day write a book called *Splash*. After all, she has always been passionate about leading the introspective from their individual reflection pools into more public ones. Over the years, I have watched her encourage the reticent to jump in and play with others on their own terms. In fact, she has been unflappable in her passion to get the reserved to go from living the lives of wallflowers to diving into their own power. In fact, with every fun but no-nonsense intervention, I have come to think of Carole as the World's Foremost Lifeguard for Introverts.

To be sure, Carole saved my life. Along with a group of friends, she staged an intervention of sorts that turned my life from inside-out to right-side-in. Up until then, I was an extrovert wannabe. I was leaking energy needlessly by trying constantly to be the big fish in ponds where I didn't even belong. With Carole's help, I was able to see that I was clearly in over my head. She helped me own the gifts of introversion and compete on my own terms. Without her gentle prodding, I might not have admitted to myself my true nature or allowed myself to do things that I have come to love to do - like sit alone and write - and then, with my batteries recharged, face the business of life with renewed confidence.

Looking back, *Splash* is not an introvert's guide to instant success where all you do is add water. After all, Carole did not promise that it would be easy, only that it would get easier for those who practice and who mindfully do things right.

Looking forward, I for one will return to this book from time to time to check in with how I am doing, and for strategies for moving ahead. I encourage you to jump in and do the same. In the meantime, enjoy the swim.

Paul Huschilt

Author, humorist, professional speaker

References

Baber, Anne, & Lynne Waymon, *Great Connections*. Manassas Park: Impact Publications, 1991

Balzano, Frederica J., Ph.D. *Why Should Extroverts Make All the Money?* Chicago: Contemporary Books, 1999

Berens, Linda V., *Understanding Yourself and Others®: An Introduction to the 4 Temperaments*. Huntington Beach: Telos Publications, 2006

Bowles, Clare, *If Only You Could Read My Mind*. Burnstown: General Store Publishing House, 2000

Byrne, Rhonda, *The Secret*. New York: Atria Books, 2006

Collins, Jim, *Good to Great*. New York: HarperCollins Publishers Inc, 2001

Demarais, Ann, Ph.D. & Valerie White, Ph.D., *First Impressions*: What You Don't Know About How Others See You. New York: Bantam Dell, 2004

Gray, John, Ph.D., *Men Are From Mars, Women Are From Venus*. New York: HarperCollins, 1992

Honeychurch, Carole, M.A., & Angela Watrous, *Talk to Me*. Oakland: New Harbinger Publications Inc., 2003

Jung, C. G., *Psychological Types*. Princeton: Princeton University Press, 1976.

Laney, Marti Olsen, Psy.D., *The Introvert Advantage*. New York: Workman Publishing Company, Inc, 2002

Laney, Marti Olsen, Psy.D. & Michael L. Laney, *The Introvert and Extrovert in Love*. Oakland: New Harbinger Publications, Inc 2007

Lowndes, Leil, *How to Talk to Anyone*. New York: McGraw-Hill, 2003

Montgomery, Stephen, Ph.D., *People Patterns*. Del Mar: Archer Publications, 2002

Prentice, Steve, *Cool-Time and the Two-Pound Bucket*. Hamilton: InstaBook, 2004

Ready, Romilla & Kate Burton, *Neuro-linguistic Programming for Dummies*. Hoboken: Wiley Pub., 2004

Reno, Tosca, B.Sc., B.Ed., *The Eat Clean Diet.* Mississauga: Robert Kennedy Pub., 2006

Shapiro, Kenneth Joel, & Irving E. Alexander, *The Experience of Introversion.* Durham: Duke University Press, 1975

Stanier, Michael Bungay, *Get Unstuck and Get Going.* Toronto: Box of Crayons Press, 2005

Usheroff, Roz, *The Leaders Edge.* West Palm Beach: The Usheroff Institute, Inc. 1999

Weir, Meghan, *Confessions of an Introvert.* Lincoln: iUniverse, 2006

Zander, Rosamund Stone, & Benjamin Zander, *The Art of Possibility.* Boston: Harvard Business School Press, 2000

Towel Off Here

Breinigsville, PA USA
12 January 2010
230637BV00002B/1/P